my GUT makes ALCOHOL

THE SCIENCE AND STORIES
OF AUTO-BREWERY SYNDROME

BARBARA CORDELL

In examining disease, we gain wisdom about anatomy and physiology and biology. In examining the person with disease, we gain wisdom about life.

— *Oliver Sacks*

FOR JOE

'Nuff said

CONTENTS

INTRODUCTION

Picture this: I was at my pastor's house for an Easter luncheon after church and I watched my husband Joe fall off the porch as if he were stone cold drunk. My gut clenched and then lurched; my heart sank, and my legs began to quiver. So many emotions went through my body-mind: shock, fear, embarrassment, worry, and confusion. I felt overwhelmed.

Joe is as dependable as the day is long. He's a compassionate nurse, wonderful husband, and faithful companion. Joe was fine all morning as we dressed, ate breakfast, and attended church. He drove to our pastor's home, we ate lunch and then out of nowhere, he turned pale, his eyes glazed over, he began slurring his words, and then he stumbled off the porch. Several of our friends helped him out of the bushes and back to standing but we all knew something was seriously wrong.

This small church in East Texas is our community, our social circle, and the well that waters our faith. Inexplicably, I felt shame and thought people would believe he was hiding alcohol. I had watched Joe go through many of these episodes at home, seemingly drunk out of the blue; but this was the first time in public among my church family.

"What is wrong with him?" "Do you think he is having a stroke?" "Does he need to go to the hospital?"

I was sure, despite our friends' compassion and concern they had thoughts of alcoholism. We coordinated getting the cars home, so Joe didn't have to drive. Part of me was mortified, but another part of me was relieved; finally, someone besides me was seeing this bizarre condition where he was drunk without drinking.

......

In the year 2010, I'd been a nurse for nearly forty years, and a doctor for twenty-one of those years, having earned a master's degree in nursing and a research-based Ph.D. in health counseling. I'd never heard the term "Auto-Brewery Syndrome" and I had no idea how much that term was about to change my life.

Joe had been having these outlandish drunken-like episodes for nearly six years and I naturally searched the academic literature to find out what could possibly be going on with him. With the first serious episode I thought he was having a stroke, but when that was ruled out, we started to believe he had a neurological problem or an endocrine blood sugar disorder – perhaps diabetes or hypoglycemia.

Joe is also a nurse and had access, then as now, to the healthcare provided by the hospital where he works. Being friends with many of the doctors, he got lots of informal consults as well as more formal testing and medical consults. None of the doctors had a clue what might be going on, but his episodes were becoming more frequent and severe.

No one ever mentioned alcohol until the day I called an ambulance for a particularly severe episode. Part of the routine testing of someone who is nearly unconscious is to test their blood alcohol level (BAC); his was a whopping .271% - over three times the legal limit in Texas. I was astounded! Joe would have to have had 11-12 drinks to test that high, but he hadn't been drinking alcohol.

Even now, it's hard for me to use the word "drunk" because that implies drinking; most of the time he had not been drinking *at all* when these symptoms came on. I was bewildered that he could suddenly become drunk. The doctors said it was impossible, but I was witnessing it firsthand so I began to search the literature for what could make someone drunk without drinking.

A dear friend, Susan Rushing, helped me research the symptoms and discovered the term Auto-Brewery Syndrome (ABS). Thus, began my journey of searching the literature for ABS; and searching, and searching. While there were only a few articles on the subject, they were enough to establish my belief that ABS was what Joe had.

After a long, strange trip through medicine at its worst - health care providers accusing us of hiding alcohol, doctors saying we must be lying, or physicians denying that something like ABS could exist - we finally found a gastroenterologist in our small town who was willing to listen to us with an open mind.

In fact, after reading the articles we took to him, Dr. Justin McCarthy diagnosed Joe with ABS. After successfully treating Joe, Dr. McCarthy suggested to me that we publish his case in the medical literature which we did in 2012.[1] I dusted off my hands thinking "that was that!"

But in September of 2013, National Public Radio (NPR) published an online blog about our case, *Auto-Brewery Syndrome: Apparently, You Can Make Beer in Your Gut*[2] in *the SALT* that went viral. While the title is not quite accurate, since ABS produces ethanol not beer, the blog brought our open source article into public awareness, with over 54,000 downloads in the first year and over 203,675 views to date.

Suddenly, I was getting emails and calls from all over the world from people who had symptoms and from people wanting to know more about this strange and interesting malady. Doctors and nurses were calling, telling me they suspected one of their patients might have ABS.

This was the beginning of a sojourn that I joke is a second full-time job in my life. I accepted every interview I was offered, from local newspapers, radio stations, TV shows, even ABC 20/20: My Strange Affliction[3] and

1   Cordell B, McCarthy J. (2013) A case study of gut fermentation syndrome (auto-brewery) with *Saccharomyces cerevisiae* as the causative organism. *Intl J Clin Med* 4:7. Article ID:33912, 4 p. Open Access: http://file.scirp.org/Html/1-2100535_33912.htm

2   National Public Radio. Auto-Brewery Syndrome: Apparently you can make beer in your gut. *The SALT* https://www.npr.org/sections/thesalt/2013/09/17/223345977/auto-brewery-syndrome-apparently-you-can-make-beer-in-your-gut

3   ABC 20/20. Auto-Brewery Syndrome: *My Strange Affliction* https://www.youtube.com/watch?v=0-hyPypkyWs. Retrieved: 11-5-18

BBC: The Human Brewery[4], most of which were very professionally done. I still have friends tell me they saw me recently on BBC, or 20/20.

A few of the radio interviewers tried to laugh and make jokes about how wonderful it was to brew your own beer in your belly, but I used every opportunity to inform and educate while trying not to be too big a killjoy. I acknowledge that it might sound funny, but to the people suffering, it's *terrible* because they never know when they might have an episode and endanger their own or someone else's life.

In time, I was getting so many calls and emails that I started a website: www.autobrewery.info and linked it to a closed Facebook support group page started by one of our treating doctors. That's when I began to understand the gravity of this condition as hundreds of people requested to join the group.

I have heard so many heart-wrenching stories by patients and family members that I've lost count. Family members freely express their worry and concern that their loved ones will hurt someone during an episode; they express depression when they cannot find effective treatment, and most distressingly, they express frustration and anger at the doctors and staff who don't believe them and are often blatantly cruel in the face of their plight.

The flip side of that, of course, is the information, support, care, love, and hope offered by members of the group to one another. Weekly I'm privileged to witness compassion and advocacy by many of our members, not just helping one another but reaching out to medical organizations, hospitals, doctors and other primary providers, nurses, chiropractors, nutritionists, and even dentists to try and get ABS recognized and treated.

I've been in touch with over 250 families affected by ABS, so I thought it was time to tell our stories. The following pages are filled with the science of what we know so far that is contributing to ABS and the stories told by people with ABS and their loved ones – the caregivers – shared in their own words.

---

4   BBC. The Human Brewery: World's Weirdest Events Episode 3 Preview (full episode available on NetFlix). https://www.youtube.com/watch?v=-cIVkJYFyuk. Retrieved 11-5-18

These stories are a small slice of the painful accounts I have heard over the past decade detailing health care provider ignorance, alarming trips to the ER, accusations of hidden alcohol consumption, harrowing descriptions of arrests and DWI convictions, and ruined marriages, finances, and lives.

I use the term "patient" throughout the book because the word comes from the Latin word *patientem* meaning "enduring or suffering" and gives us the word "patience". Several decades ago, the nursing profession attempted to substitute the word "client" for "patient", and it did not stick. I'm glad. I've grown to appreciate the word patient because of what those with ABS endure.

While I touch on the aspects of diagnosis and treatment of Auto-Brewery Syndrome, this book is in no way intended to substitute for medical advice from a primary provider who conducts a thorough assessment. The names of some of the patients and caregivers have been changed to protect their privacy.

My purpose in writing this book is a call to action. I'm challenging healthcare providers to listen to patients who don't fit the usual mold. And I'm asking all of us to be more compassionate toward anyone with a rare or invisible illness.

Please check out my website at www.autobrewery.info. Whether you are looking for personal or professional guidance or just a good read, I hope you absorb the science and learn from our stories.

CHAPTER 1 ~

A MEDICAL SCOTOMA

Medicine is a science of Uncertainty and an art of Probability

— *Sir William Osler, Founder of Johns Hopkins Hospital*

Imagine it's a weekday morning and you get dressed and drive to work like you do every day, but later your co-workers report you are passed out in your car. Somehow, you made the drive from home to the parking lot, but never made it inside the office. You feel unmoored, adrift with no explanation, and no way to make it back to the harbor. That's the experience of ABS.

One of the patients in our support group, Mark, who doesn't drink alcohol at all, describes his episodes this way: *I don't feel a flare coming on. I feel okay and think everything is fine, but then I realize I'm impaired. I can't move or do a simple math problem; then when I talk, someone tells me I'm not making sense. I check my BAC and find it's .04 to .09. After that, I'm in a daze until I come back down. My hangovers last 2-3 days with malaise, lots of gas and burping. Then the cycle starts all over again.*

Auto-Brewery Syndrome (ABS) is an ailment whereby patients become intoxicated without ingesting alcohol and the vast majority of doctors in the U.S. have never heard of it. The underlying mechanism is an overgrowth of yeast somewhere in the gut that ferments carbohydrates into alcohol. Beyond that initial understanding, we have mountains to scale in order to discover the how and why of the malady, not to mention how to treat it.

We all like to believe that science is neat and tidy, and that it has the answers to all our sicknesses. After all, we have nano-technology, gene therapy, and microsurgery; we've solved so many medical mysteries! But the truth is, medical diagnosis and decision-making is still messy and uncertain, the science is incomplete, and not all health providers practice with the same rigor and ethics.

In his posthumously published book *The River of Consciousness*, Dr. Oliver Sacks aptly describes the collective phenomena of forgetting, resisting, or ignoring previous scientific work as "cultural or historical scotomas".[5] He states, "Scotoma, surprisingly common in all fields of science…involves a loss of knowledge, a forgetting of insights that once seemed clearly established, and sometimes a regression to less perceptive explanations" (p.205).

Neurologists use the term scotoma to mean a "disconnection or hiatus in perception, essentially a gap in consciousness produced by a neurological lesion." A mental scotoma in psychiatry is a figurative blind spot in a person's psychological awareness, the patient being unable to gain insight into and to understand his mental problems; a lack of insight.

A medical scotoma, then, could be viewed as a loss of seeing or perceiving, or even ignoring what has been described, historically documented, and shared in the medical literature. ABS is a scotoma on a long list of medical scotomas. A scotoma is literally a blind spot in an otherwise normal visual field but is figuratively a blind spot caused by skepticism, prematurity, forgetting or even bias.

SKEPTICISM

Scientists are trained to conceive a hypothesis and then set about disproving the hypothesis; we start with what is known and then move into new territory. All research methods are developed to minimize bias and eliminate the possibility of chance. Therefore, the scientific method predisposes researchers to be skeptics.

It's no wonder then, when a new phenomenon is first identified and described, it is often met with skepticism in the science community because it

---

5   Sacks O. (2017) The River of Consciousness. New York: Alfred A. Knopf

doesn't fit neatly into the current belief structure. We cling to what we know from research and experience.

Culture is replete with examples playing out in public discourse where we ignore data and even jeopardize human lives with our denial. At times scientists face denial of data even when they show the public their overwhelming evidence. Climate scientists face this issue when people deny that climate change exists, even when presented with the overwhelming evidence from 98% of all scientists world-wide who study the earth's climate.

Medical practitioners are not immune to being skeptical of data, but often if new information doesn't change the behavior of clinicians, it can be dangerous to the lives of patients. Sometimes we researchers feel like Louis Pasteur who met with great disbelief for his theory of the cause of disease from microbes at a time when most of the scientific world believed in spontaneous generation.

I sometimes feel like humans naturally resist change and new ideas; even though science tells me (ha!) we only resist what we believe is not in our best interest. We must ask, why would a doctor think that knowing about ABS is not in his or her best interest? It's certainly not in the best interest of his or her patients.

PREMATURITY

Another way a medical syndrome is a scotoma is through prematurity; a health problem is identified before the science can explain it. An example of prematurity is Sudden Infant Death Syndrome, or SIDS. Up to the 1990s medical practitioners and others believed a baby was accidentally enveloped and suffocated by the mother or evil spirits.[6]

By the early 1900s most infants were in separate cots and the blame shifted from the mothers to suffocation by soft pillows and blankets. But

---

6   Russell-Jones D. (1985) Sudden infant death in history and literature. *Arch Dis in Childhood* 60:278-281. http://dx.doi.org/10.1136/adc.60.3.278

with the advent of WWII and improved pathology, the autopsies frequently cited "natural causes" for the infant deaths.

Any other explanation of SIDS was non-existent until the 1960s when the World Health Organization took notice and began funding conferences and research into the causes of SIDS. By the 2000s, evidence showed SIDS was linked to abnormalities in the brainstem, a part of the brain that helps control heart rate, breathing, blood pressure, temperature, and arousal.[7]

This evidence was premature, however, as it was another decade before medical science developed enough of a structure and the technology to test the theory of a brainstem link to SIDS. In 2010, Dr. John Duncan discovered a link of a brain enzyme (5-HT disorder) deficiency[8] which supports the theory of a problem with regulation of vital functions such as breathing in these babies.

Researchers continue to study tissue samples of babies who die unexplained deaths to discover the cause, and more importantly to try and prevent the nearly 4,000 SIDS deaths each year in the U.S. The mechanism of SIDS is *still unknown*, but no one ever denied that infants were dying mysterious deaths. At least in the 21st century, the medical establishment is finally able to determine possible underlying causes.

FORGETTING

If a disease is rare, it is likely to be overlooked or forgotten by the medical community. Especially if the previous literature is older or obscure, or published in other countries less respected by U.S. doctors. Some rare diseases are lucky to find a celebrity to shine a spotlight on the disorder to raise funds, or a benefactor who cares about the cause and privately funds research. Barring those windfalls, federal funds are scarce to research rare diseases, especially ones like ABS with so many skeptics.

---

7   McEntire B. (2018) National SIDS Act of 1974. https://sids.org/about-us/sids-historical-perspective/

8   Duncan J, Paterson D, Hoffman J, et al. (2010) Brainstem serotonergic deficiency in sudden infant death syndrome. *JAMA* 303(5): 430-437

Even the incredibly prevalent disease of alcoholism is underfunded due to a common forgetfulness that it is a medical disease and not a failure of will power. Even physicians forget data and fall prey to common misconceptions. Our biases could contribute to forgetting and scientists may spend a lifetime trying to remind their colleagues of data based on research.

AN EXAMPLE OF SCOTOMA

What if you lost your right arm in an accident and dreamed it was still there? When you awake, you feel tingling, and then pain. You swear it's still there! But when you look, the arm is gone, and you remember the accident and the surgery to repair the stump. You remember the conversation with the doctor who reassured you a great prognosis with a prosthesis. But your right arm is on fire with pain; in fact, it's excruciating.

Phantom limb syndrome is residual sensory experience after the patient has lost a limb. Pain, itching, and tingling all continue even though there is no body part to send those messages back to the brain. The history of phantom limb provides a great example of all three aspects of medical scotoma: skepticism, prematurity, and forgetting.

French surgeon Ambroise Paré first described phantom limb in 1552. His wounded soldiers complained of pain in their amputated limbs, which he termed "deceptive sensations." In 1642, French scientist, mathematician, and philosopher René Descartes published the same syndrome as did others during this 90-year period.

The skepticism during these days lodged on an idea that phantom limb was a "psychological problem" caused by grief and the desire to believe the limb was still present. Many also believed sensations from nerve endings could deceive the brain into an unreal conclusion.

Descartes stated that "much of what comes in through the senses is obscure and confused. This deception of the senses is natural... In countless such cases I found that the judgments of the external senses were mistaken, and the same was true of the internal senses." [9]

The information on phantom limb was then largely overlooked, or forgotten because, over 150 years later, German physician Aaron Lemos published his doctoral dissertation on "The Continuing Pain of an Amputated Limb" without citing any of the numerous previously published reports.[10] Was he not aware of the published articles? Did he not have access to an academic library? Or did he conveniently, or even truly, forget?

And the concept was certainly premature. It wasn't until the early 1800s that scientists connected phantom limb to ideas about nerves, the brain, sensory perception, and ultimately proprioception.[11] The contemporaneous study of physiology enlightened the doctors and the concept of a neurological explanation was finally plausible.

But even then, scientists and clinicians kept forgetting. In 1864, Silas Weir Mitchell, a neurologist during the American Civil War wrote a special circular issued by the surgeon general's office and was the first to use the term "phantom limb" in a publication in 1871.[12] His observations were not replicated and all but disappeared until the syndrome was "re-discovered" during World War I. French neurologist Joseph Babinski, apparently forgetting or intentionally ignoring the prior mentioned work, published a report in 1917.

Babinski's writing on phantom limb seems to have been forgotten as well because, during World War II, Soviet neurologists published a book on rehabilitation which included a vivid description of phantom limb symptoms with no reference to either Babinski or Mitchell.[13]

---

9   Finger S, Hustwit M. (2003) Five early accounts of phantom limb in context: Pare, Descartes, Lemos, Bell, and Mitchell. *Neurosurgery* 52(3):685-676

10   Finger, Ibid

11   Van Gijn J. (2003) Charles Bell (1774-1842). *J Neur* 258:1189-1190. https://link.springer.com/content/pdf/10.1007/s00415-011-5912-5.pdf

12   Sacks, Ibid

13   Rugnetta M. (2018) Phantom Limb Syndrome. https://www.britannica.com/science/phantom-limb-syndrome

Once again, the work on phantom limb descended into oblivion. The concept of phantom limb pain was finally revived and confirmed as a neurological experience during more recent wars in Vietnam, Afghanistan, and Syria, and is now firmly ensconced in the medical literature about amputation and rehabilitation.

Ambroise Paré penned, "Verily it is a thing wondrous strange and prodigious, and which will scarce be credited, unless by such as have seene with their eyes, and heard with their ears the Patients…".

••••••

I clearly see how early examples of medical scotoma might be partially blamed on the lack of ease of communication of scientific data. Prior to the advent of the Internet, finding, let alone sharing scientific information was a hit and miss proposition. Only the largest and finest libraries could house current scientific information and they were few and far between. But today, a medical scotoma can no longer be blamed on lack of available information.

How then, with instant access to the huge body of scientific literature, can physicians continue to be blind to what is clearly in front of them? Some people get drunk without drinking. Is it a collective forgetting? Or is the information on ABS still premature? Or does the medical culture have entrenched biases about alcohol that makes doctors skeptical?

The literature contains numerous case studies of ABS, yet even when we present such examples to physicians, we are often met with statements such as "that's impossible," and "no such thing exists." Perhaps doctors believe it's not in their best interest to embrace a rare and weird syndrome. Or maybe they must see it with their own eyes.

I introduce the concept of scotoma so forcefully because collectively, this is where we are when it comes to ABS. We in the ABS support community feel we are being denied, forgotten, and in some cases, punished. Every one of us, at one point or another, heard the words, "I've never heard of this," or "No one gets drunk without drinking."

When I first found the term ABS, I explained it to a friend of mine who is an ER doctor. I asked if he would be willing to read the articles I found to see if ABS is what Joe might have. He said, "That's bullshit. There's no way the body can't make alcohol and besides, it's not my area." What hubris it takes to admit something is not your area of expertise, and still declare it impossible.

••••••

The medical establishment often feels like a fraternity whose beliefs are so entrenched that only a few brave souls dare challenge the status quo. I remember many times in my career when I challenged doctors with science. While educating patients was always rewarding, the interactions with doctors often showed me how closed-minded they could be.

One surgeon tried to get me fired for educating a patient about the surgery he was going to have the next morning. The frightened man started the conversation with, "I have to have surgery tomorrow," and I said, "You are in charge of what happens to your body and you can choose to have the surgery or not." He was surprised, eager to listen, and asked many questions.

I spent nearly an hour educating that gentleman about open-heart surgery and the risks and long-term outcomes of the procedure based on the latest research. I shared the medical treatment options available to him in lieu of surgery and he told me he would think it over. The patient told the doctor the next morning that he'd decided not to have the surgery. Man was that doctor mad! Do you think the doctor was concerned about the best interest of the patient? Or perhaps his own self-interest in his reputation and his income?

HORSES VS. ZEBRAS

When teaching medical students to weigh medical evidence, the aphorism of "horses versus zebras" is intended as a caution against biases. A *zebra* is the medical slang for an unexpected, rare, or exotic diagnosis and *horses* denotes the more common, everyday maladies.

Dr. Theodore Woodward, a professor at the University of Maryland School of Medicine, is credited with having coined the term, circa 1950, by saying, "When you hear hoofbeats, think of horses, not zebras." The maxim is now intended to help diagnosticians arrive at a differential diagnosis by looking first for the more common explanation and only later for the rare or surprising diagnosis.

According to Dr. John Sotos, a cardiologist trained at Johns Hopkins University School of Medicine, only medical novices are predisposed to make rare diagnoses because of (a) "the more easily remembered are judged more probable" and (b) "the striking and the novel stay longer in the mind".[14]

It's no wonder the experienced physicians rarely get past the very common thought that someone who is drunk must have been drinking. Since Auto-Brewery Syndrome is not a zebra but a duck-billed platypus, most providers think we are confabulating.

OUR SCOTOMA

In the 1950s to 1970s, Japanese doctors authored multiple cases describing Auto-Brewery Syndrome, and named it "drunken disease".[15,16] During the 1980s and 90s, an assembly of doctors and nutritionists in England, Keith Eaton, Adrian Hunnisett, and John McLaren Howard published numerous

---

14   Sotos J. (2006) [1991] Zebra Cards: An Aid to Obscure Diagnoses. Mt. Vernon, VA: Mt. Vernon Book Systems. ISBN 978-0-9818193-0-3

15   Iwata K. (1972) A review of the literature on drunken syndromes due to yeasts in the gastrointestinal tract. *Int Spec Symp Yeast* Tokyo: University of Tokyo Press: 260-8

16   Kaji H, Asanuma Y, Ide H, et al. (1976) The Auto-Brewery Syndrome – the repeated attacks of alcoholic intoxication due to the overgrowth of *Candida (albicans)* in the gastrointestinal tract. *Materia Medica Polona* 4(29):429-435

articles on ABS.[17,18,19,20] They acted quite unsurprised that the syndrome existed in Great Britain and even called it an "old condition".

Now the British medical system has forgotten their own history. I receive frequent calls and emails from UK patients desperate for help who were turned away by their doctors. Like the U.S., Auto-Brewery Syndrome is rare enough that it only poses an occasional challenge to the neat little physiology the Brits have come to believe about alcohol, intoxication, and addiction.

Western medicine hardly acknowledges the syndrome, and most doctors have never even heard of it, which is why I believe ABS is seriously under-diagnosed. Barely a week goes by that I'm not contacted by a person who believes he, she or a loved one has ABS.

Dr. Brian Welch and colleagues, from none other than Mayo Clinic, report a case of Auto-Brewery Syndrome but then state, "clinical consideration of 'auto-brewery' should be undertaken with substantial caution given the lack of validated mechanisms linking endogenous ethanol production to peripheral blood ethanol."[21] Since when do we require 'validated mechanisms' before diagnosing a disease? And what the heck does that even mean?

Diabetes was first described in 250 BCE. For centuries, no one understood an underlying cause for diabetes, but that didn't stop diagnosis, documentation, and attempted treatment of the affliction. During the 1800s and early 1900s, physicians noted that dietary changes could improve diabetes, but it wasn't until 1920 that insulin was first administered. Dr. Frederick Banting

---

17   Hunnisett A, Howard J. (1990) Gut fermentation (or the 'auto-brewery') syndrome: A new clinical test with initial observations and discussion of clinical and biochemical implications. *J Nutr Med* 1(1):33-39

18   Eaton K. (1991) Gut fermentation: a reappraisal of an old clinical condition with diagnostic tests and management: discussion paper. *J Royal Soc Med* 84:669-71

19   Eaton K, Howard M, Hunnisett A. (1994) Urinary beta-alanine excretion is a marker of abnormal as well as normal gut fermentation. *J Nutr Med* 4(2):157-163

20   Eaton K, Howard M, Howard J. (1995) Gut permeability measured by polyethylene glycol absorption in abnormal gut fermentation as compared with food intolerance. *J Royal Soc Med* 88:63-66

21   Welch B, Prabhu N, Walkoff L, Trenkner S. (2016) Auto-Brewery Syndrome in the setting of long-standing Crohn's disease: A case report and review of literature. *J of Crohn's and Colitis* DOI: https://doi.org/10.1093/ecco-jcc/jjw098

of Canada and his collaborators tested insulin on animals and finally tried insulin on a diabetic patient, earning a Nobel prize in Medicine in 1923.[22,23]

SIDS, phantom limb, diabetes, and many other diseases and syndromes required years, decades or even centuries to propose a theory, let alone validate an underlying mechanism or cause. Just because we don't understand something does not mean it should be denied and ignored.

And in fact, an underlying mechanism for ABS has been proposed by de Medeiros and de Lima.[24] In studying the question of non-alcoholic fatty liver disease (NAFLD), they hypothesize that NAFLD may be caused by endogenous alcohol. De Medeiros and de Lima base their theory on numerous studies of people who produce higher levels of endogenous ethanol (EE). They cite multiple factors and studies including those of ABS linked to endogenous alcohol as well as gut-derived bacterial toxins to conclude their belief in the hypothesis.

••••••

The institutional denial and forgetting continues; many doctors refuse even to entertain the notion of looking at ABS. Sadly, we in the Auto-Brewery community have had to demand that physicians and other primary providers see with their own eyes the patient's "signs and symptoms" and lab tests before they become believers. Only a handful of our providers are even willing to look and be the inquisitive and open-minded scientists that all doctors should be.

---

22   History of Diabetes. https://www.everydayhealth.com/diabetes/understanding/diabetes-mellitus-through-time.aspx Retrieved on 8-16-18

23   Lakhtakia R. (2013) The History of Diabetes Mellitus. *Sultan Qaboos Univ Med J* 13(3):368-370. PMID: 23984020

24   De Medeiros I, de Lima J. (2015) Is nonalcoholic fatty liver disease an endogenous alcoholic fatty liver disease? – A mechanistic hypothesis. *Medical Hypotheses* 85:148-152. https://doi.org/10.1016/j.mehy.2015.04.021

I believe our emerging knowledge of the microbiome will explode our understanding of ABS in the coming years. Meanwhile, how do we continue to shed light on a misunderstood, underdiagnosed, denied and forgotten rare syndrome?

CITIZEN SCIENTISTS

One of the ways under-studied diseases eventually come to light is through the work of family members. Dr. Isaac Kohane, chair of the Department of Biomedical Informatics at Harvard Medical School describes family members who know medicine does not have good answers for their loved ones, as "biomedical citizen science leaders." He asserts:

> no one feels the urgency to find the answer as much as they do, and they will pour all their free time…to both master the science and serve as general scientific contractor to coordinate all the experts and groups they have engaged. They are…the scientific quarterback without brakes.[25]

We in the ABS community have gathered an amazing assembly of *biomedical citizen science leaders* who spend countless hours searching the literature, discussing possible symptoms and treatments, and supporting one another. Anger over being dismissed fuels much of our activism.

Family members express frustration at the unwillingness of so many primary providers (mostly physicians) to listen to what they are saying. A typical quote is: *If the doctors thought this was a 'real' condition we could get cultures done-- but we can't even get them to listen. 'Here's your brochure on alcoholism, don't let the door hit you on the way out' has been the result of our doctor and hospital visits.*

---

25   Kohane I. (2017) Medical science should learn to tap the urgency of families desperate to save loved ones. http://www.wbur.org/commonhealth/2017/12/08/families-citizen-scientists

Here's another post from one of the most active advocates in our support group:

Michelle: *I just want to remind you all that if you have a doctor that has turned you away and was dismissive regarding ABS, please reach out to me with the doctor's name, address and Email address (preferred).*

I have sent emails regarding ABS on behalf of people in this group to their doctors to bring awareness of ABS and have offered those doctors a chance to read some documentation on ABS and *encouraged them to reach out to our NY doctors.*

Please do not accept "no" for an answer. Just collect their information and send it to me. I live in an area where we have every possible major medical institution at our fingertips and we were turned away by the best of the best - I did not accept no for an answer, and neither should you.

I have every intention of getting ABS on the map, and I will continue to make waves.

Most importantly, our citizen leaders channel their anger and frustration into advocacy for patients even when they or their family member has eliminated their symptoms. They contact physicians, try to disseminate information, and help one another prepare for doctor visits to ensure they are not summarily dismissed. Together we are stronger than we ever thought we could be. Someday, we will put this medical scotoma ABS on the map again, this time to stay.

CHAPTER 2

FASCINATING FERMENTATION

...fermentation puts us in touch with the ever-present tug, in life, of death.

— *Michael Pollan, Cooked*

People with Auto-Brewery Syndrome teeter on the brink between healthy digestion and one or two fermenting yeast organisms growing wildly out of control like kudzu on the banks of southern highways. Amazingly, so much of our health and life takes place on an invisible plane of microbial activity that we must study microbes to understand ABS.

Microorganisms such as bacteria and yeast mostly serve as decomposers and guardians in our air, in the soil, on our skin, and in our bodies. To understand health and disease related to ABS, let's peer into a microscope and examine some of those infinitesimal microbes specifically, those that ferment.

FERMENTATION IN NATURE

Eventually all organic matter breaks down by the process of fermentation through the enzymatic action of bacteria, molds, and yeasts. We can usually smell the odor of decomposition as biological material such as leaves, or dead animals begins to decay. This degradation is going on constantly all around us; for example, in the soil. Initially in your compost pile, you smell putrefaction, but later, the pile turns to nutrient-rich soil for your garden that smells refreshed and renewed.

If you open your refrigerator you may encounter the wonderful beginnings of fermentation in items such as yogurt, vinegar, or sauerkraut. You may also see and smell the further result of fermentation, known as rotting, when you discover a forgotten leftover that turned green and fuzzy, or the lettuce that turned to brown liquid.

Technically, fermentation is a metabolic process that consumes sugar in the absence of oxygen. The end products of fermentation by yeast, bacteria, and even human oxygen-starved muscle cells are organic acids, gases, or alcohol.

FERMENTATION OF FOOD

The variety of fermenting processes and resulting food and drink is breathtaking. We consume fermented food daily even as part of a typical Western diet. Milk, cheese, vinegar, olives, soy sauce, and other fermented foodstuffs grace our plates and cups on a regular basis.

Humans began the intentional transformation of food known as fermentation, over 12,000 years ago. Fermentation assisted the meteoric rise in the number of people on the planet by allowing people to preserve and store food for future days instead of eating only what they killed or harvested on the same day.

Along with farming and rudimentary tools, fermenting food helped humans take a giant leap forward into the New Stone Age after centuries of only having fire. In addition to preservation, fermentation had the magical ability to make otherwise inedible foods edible, to add flavor and nutritional value, and to decrease toxicity.

One of the earliest identifications of fermented food was in the Neolithic period around 10,000 BCE and included beer, wine, leavened bread, and cheese.[26] These early human fermenters dug holes into the earth and lined the cavity with leaves. They then added solid food and covered it with dirt where the temperature was cool and constant. They put liquids into animal skins or primitive crocks before placing them into the hollow.

An early Mesolithic site in Sweden indicates the people living there around 7000 BCE fermented fish in pits in the ground. Earthenware jars in Northern China revealed that between 7000 and 6600 BCE, the people living there fermented an alcoholic beverage made from rice, honey, and hawthorne fruit.[27]

The early Chinese inoculated food with molds (which we now know produce enzymes), to create products like miso, tofu, and soy sauce.[28,29] Most likely, they added salt to some foods which encouraged certain natural microorganisms to ferment and inhibit spoilage, resulting in nutritious and longer lasting foodstuff.

Salting, smoking, and freezing later joined fermentation as food preservation. But only fermentation carried the mysterious trait of metamorphosing the food or drink into something that tasted, smelled, and felt entirely different.

Early human cultures revered the conversion of food through fermentation as a mysterious act of divine intervention - which is quite understandable in the absence of a scientific explanation. The Egyptians and Greeks

26   Terefe N. (2016) Food fermentation. *Reference Module in Food Sciences* http://dx.doi.org/10.1016/B978-0-08-100596-5.03420-x

27   Bourdichon F, Casaregola S, Farrokh C, et al. (2011) Food fermentation: Microorganisms with technological beneficial use. *Intern Jour of Food Micro* DOI: 10.1016/j.ijfoodmicro.2011.12.030

28   Batt C. (2016) Microbiology of fermentations. *Reference Module in Food Sciences* http://dx.doi.org/10.1016/B978-0-08-100596-5.03443-0

29   Talon R, Zagorec M. (2017) Beneficial microorganisms for food manufacturing- fermented and biopreserved foods and beverages. *Microorganisms* 5(71). DOI: 10.3390/microorganisms5040071

named gods for beer and wine, and the Japanese dedicated shrines to miso and shoyu.

Imagine what strange flavors and textures early people must have discovered -- and how brave those first persons must have been to try each of these miraculous or horrible new foods! Food fermentation is a microcosm of life itself and runs the gamut from delectable when all goes well to putrid when something goes wrong. Like life, fermentation is biodiversity in action and our lives would surely be diminished without it.

••••••

In our long dalliance with this magical process, scientists with microscopes untangled the extensive web of the fermentation process and its microbic contributors. Food fermentation is a living process whereby microorganisms of bacteria and yeast devour the food and transform it into a nourishment poles apart; think cabbage to sauerkraut. The result is often a pungent, sour, funky but edible substance on the very edge of rot.

Intentional fermentation today continues to provide a variety of foods for most of the world's population, estimated to be between 20 and 40%,[30] especially in developing countries and the Far East. However, fermentation lost favor in most of the West with the advent of refrigeration, the notion that "fresh is better," and of course, our love affair with the taste and texture of sugar and fat.

The industrial revolution then promoted processed and pre-cooked convenience foods that won over our palates and our time management. Who has room left for fermented foods after all the refined foods we typically eat?

---

30   Wang J, Fung D. (2008) Alkaline-fermented foods: A review with emphasis on pidan fermentation. *Critical Reviews in Microbiology* 22:2, 101-138. https://doi.org/10.3109/10408419609106457

Now though, with the emerging science about the health of the gut and its connection to auto-immune disorders, brain function, and mood disorders, food fermentation is regaining popularity in the West. Health practitioners promote fermented foods such as kefir, kombucha, and sauerkraut for health and wellness, as well as a mechanism to ingest "natural" probiotics. Wellness practitioners and many popular books espouse this new food revolution.

Michael Pollan, in his incredibly fascinating book *Cooked,* describes a fermenting underground -- impassioned "post-Pasteurians" who act outside the norms of U.S. society. In fact, they break laws by drinking unpasteurized milk. But they continue using wild cultures and spreading their deeply held political and ecological philosophy.[31] These fermenters zealously profess a cult-like doctrine through farmers' markets, websites, and best-selling books. To be fair, fermented foods do make us feel good on so many levels – even high!

• • • • • •

Three broad categories of microbial food fermentation traditionally used throughout history are: lactic acid, alkaline, and fungal fermentation.[32]

Lactic acid fermentation creates delightful foods such as sausage, cheese, yogurt, sauerkraut and kimchi. In the process of lactic acid fermentation, glucose, six-carbon sugars, and disaccharides of six-carbon sugars such as lactose or sucrose are metabolized into energy at the cellular level and the by-product is lactate. Image 1 shows a representation of this process.

31   Pollan M. (2013) *Cooked: A Natural History of Transformation* New York: The Penguin Press

32   Duina A, Miller M, Keeney J. (2014) Budding yeast for budding geneticists: A primer on the *Saccharomyces cerevisiae* model system. *Genetics* 197:33-48. https://doi.org/10.1534/genetics.114.163188

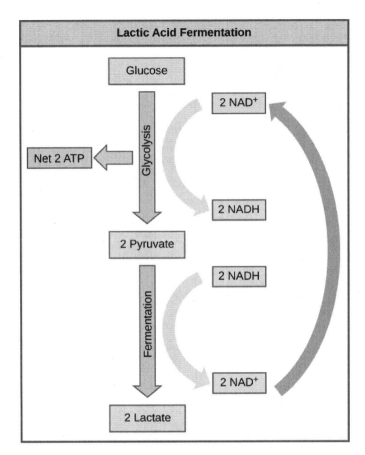

Image 1: Chemical representation of Lactic Acid Fermentation

Provided by: OpenStax CNX: Located at: http://cnx.org/contents/185cbf87-c72e-48f5-b51e-fl4f2lb5eabd@10.8. License: CC: by Attribution.

Alkaline-fermented foods are widely consumed in Southeast Asia and African countries. For example, Japanese natto, and kinema are made from cooked soybeans, dawadawa from African locust beans, ogiri from melon seeds, and pidan from fresh poultry eggs.[33]

To the Western palate, these foods are very stinky and are certainly an acquired taste. Mixed bacteria cultures principally dominated by *Bacillus subtilis,* spontaneously produce most of these foods. Alkaline fermentation is

---

33   Wang, Ibid.

a complex microbiologic process represented in Image 2, that decomposes proteins and increases the pH values to at least 7 and up to 9 (alkaline). The resulting peptides, amino acids and ammonia are what result in the putrid, strong ammoniacal odor.

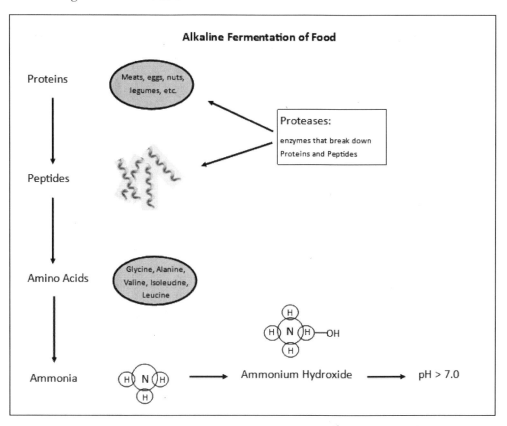

Image 2: Alkaline Fermentation of Food: By author

Yeast fermentations are the third category and the most important fermentations to understanding ABS. Yeasts generate many foods we love. Close your eyes and enter the bakery of your mind to smell that blissful loaf of sourdough bread baking. How could anyone not crave a warm fresh slice? No wonder zealous fermenters are zealot-y when they can produce such yummy indulgence in a loaf.

Sourdough starters usually contain the important yeast *Saccharomyces cerevisiae* that ferments alcohol, combined with lactic acid fermenters; either *Lactobacillus plantarum* or *Lactobacillus sanfranciscensis*. Can you guess where that last species was discovered?

The carbon dioxide bubbles created during alcohol fermentation give the bread its airy texture, and the alcohol provides the magnificent 'sour' taste so distinctive and cherished in sourdough breads. In this case, salt is used to inhibit fermentation and to toughen the gluten to hold more CO_2 which adds more rise to the dough.[34] The result is marvelous.

Few fermented foods are created by using only one species. Yeast sub-species are combined with lactic-acid ferments to produce foods such as kefir, kombucha, soy sauce, and tempeh. These combination fermentations are gaining popularity as super foods believed to promote health and healing.

• • • • • •

Natural fermentation relies on wild strains of microbes living on the vegetables, or in the air, or even on the wooden spoon or crock used. Commercial fermentation, on the other hand, uses sterile instruments in a sterile environment and counts on the introduction of a "starter culture" of microbes that has been pasteurized so that only the intended microbes reach the food.

Cheese invites us to taste the difference. The commercial varieties we buy in most chain grocery stores are bland and almost tasteless compared to the small batch artisanal cheeses burgeoning in specialty stores and farmers' markets. If you haven't done a taste comparison with your favorite type of cheese, you really should.

There is, as you might imagine, an ongoing lively debate of "natural vs. pasteurized." Laws in the U.S. are firmly on the side of Pasteurists. No doubt, pasteurization has saved many lives by standardizing a process to eliminate

---

34   Sieuwerts S, Bron P, Smid E. (2017) Mutually stimulating interactions between lactic acid bacteria in *Saccharomyces cerevisiae* in sourdough fermentation. *Food Science and Technology* https://doi.org/10.1016/j. lwt.2017.12.022

harmful bacteria that may concomitantly grow during the natural process of fermentation. Careless fermenters can cause illness and death.

Naturalists argue that pasteurization also removes the beneficial microbes that help us maintain gut health. They correctly believe if one is attentive with the natural process, the fermenting microbes will eliminate the harmful ones through competition and will maintain the beneficial ones. Diligence with the natural process also amplifies the flavor as I hope you have experienced. So, it pays to get to know and trust your fermenter.

For more on this fascinating subject, read Michael Pollan's account in *Cooked* of Benedictine Sister Noëlla Marcellino and her handmade cheese in a wooden barrel from an ancient recipe. She used science to receive dispensation from the health inspector to continue selling cheese using her natural process.

Tea is a great example of just how confusing the term fermentation can be and how different microbes produce different results. All true tea starts from the same plant: *camellia sinensis*. Black, yellow, green, oolong, and white tea are classified based on the degree of fermentation; enzymatic oxidation that is, through a crush/tear or maceration process. Even though this is considered fermentation, it's not "true" fermentation.

True microbially fermented teas include Pu-erh (with over 1,000 different microbes changing it), Anhua dark tea (not to be confused with black tea) and dozens of others.[35] The most famous yeast fermented tea, requiring sugar to ferment, is Kombucha. Even then, this true fermentation is not usually what we commonly consider fermentation because we generally think of fermentation as producing alcohol.

GOD IS GOODE

Of course, many people's favorite yeast-fermented treat is ethanol or alcohol in the form of whiskey, wine, or beer. This is the essence of our ABS

---

35   Zhang Y. Skaar I, Sulyok M, et al. (2016) The microbiome and metabolites in fermented Pu-erh tea. *PLOS* https://doi.org/10.1371/journal.pone.0157847

story as we realize several strains of yeast turn sugars into ethanol in the body as well as in the still, barrel, or cask. So, let's look at how this works.

Distilled beverages, such as whiskey and scotch, involve yeast fermentation of the "mash" coupled with a distillation process in a still to produce the alcoholic spirits. Wine and beer are direct fermentation: plant material to alcohol by yeast, mostly *Saccharomyces cerevisiae* with occasional blends of lactic acid bacilli. In fact, the original yeast was thought to come from grapes and can still be found in vineyards in abundance.[36]

Here's where the art of winemaking comes in. Vintners have an array of decisions to make selecting growing regions as well as deciding when to harvest the grapes, and whether to add yeast or allow the natural yeast to work its enchantment. The same is true with the decisions about hops for varieties of beer.

So colossal is our passion for wine and beer, that the most widely studied yeast in the world is *Saccharomyces cerevisiae*. Scientists sequenced its entire genome even before the human genome! I had no idea how important this yeast was until my husband Joe developed Auto-Brewery Syndrome from its overgrowth in his gut.

There are thousands of books and websites devoted to brewing beer. A quick Google search for "brewing beer" returned 2,480,000 hits and a search for "books on beer fermentation" garnered 472,000 results. Since the fermentation of beer helps us understand Auto-Brewery Syndrome, I'll explore it in that context; plus, it's fun and interesting.

••••••

For most of history, brewers transferred their cultures from one batch of brew to the next, called "backslopping." In the early days of beer fermentation, the foam was understood to start new brewing batches, but exactly how, was a mystery. So magical was the foaming potion burbling on the surface

---

36   Duina, Ibid

of the concoction, it was called "Godisgoode" by the brewers in medieval England. We now know that Godisgoode is really the yeast *Saccharomyces*.

The celebrated, *Saccharomyces cerevisiae*, is more commonly known as Baker's or Brewer's yeast and is actually a fungus or mold. In 1838, the German chemist Franz Meyen gave it the scientific name derived from Latin and Latinized Greek: *Saccaron-* meaning "sugar," m*yces* meaning "yeast," and *cerevisiae* meaning "of beer." [37]

When science was applied to the brewing industry in the 1800s, brewers learned how to purify yeast and control temperature and storage for more reliable-tasting beer. At the Carlsberg Brewery, a chemist named Emil Christian Hansen studied ale and lager and was able to isolate yeast from the sediments.

He cultured two species isolates: *Saccharomyces cerevisiae* from the ale and *Saccharomyces carlsbergensis* from the lager.[38] It appears the brewery claimed his discovery and got to name the yeast, or it might have been *Saccharomyces hansensis*.

As a side note, *S. cerevisiae,* has become quite a star in the biology laboratories throughout the world over the last fifty years. It turns out, once the genome was sequenced in 1996, the little organism provided a perfect medium for gene regulation studies as well as protein and amino acid studies.

Dr. Brigida Gallone and her colleagues in Belgium sequenced and determined phenotypes of 157 strains of *S. cerevisiae* yeasts used in the industry to produce beer, wine, bread, spirits, sake and bioethanol.[39] They realized all 157 yeasts originated from only five domesticated ancestors.

---

37   Livens S. (2016) Beer: Fermentation. *Encyclopedia of Food and Health* http://dx.doi.org/10.1016/B978-0-12-384947-2.00059-3

38   Greig D, Leu J. (2009) Natural history of budding yeast. *Curr Biol* 19:R886-R890

39   Gallone B, Steensels J, Troels P. (2016) Domestication and divergence of *Saccharomyces cerevisiae* beer yeasts. *Cell* http://dx.doi.org/10.1016/j.cell.2016.08.020

The five clades, or branches on the tree of life, include only two families of beer yeasts! The other three are Asian yeasts: sake yeast, win yeasts, and a mixed clade that contains bread and other yeasts. Isn't it stunning that in the whole world every brewer uses descendants of the same two families of yeast to produce beer?

The authors discovered the two dominant beer yeasts have a common ancestor as recently as 1573-1671. This suggests that people were domesticating yeast prior to the discovery of microbes. I would be fascinated to know how that worked.

Modern breweries now carefully culture, measure, and purify strains of Brewer's yeast to use in their process to produce safe and consistent-tasting beers. And much like other fermentations, beer brewing is enjoying a revival of craft-brewing and home-brewing much closer to the natural ancient traditions. The next time I have a cold one in the heat of our Texas summer, I'll remember to call it Godisgoode!

DIGESTION IN HUMANS

Most people don't realize the human gastrointestinal system, the gut, is also a fermentation powerhouse. The microbes in our guts, including the stomach, small intestines, and large intestines, are providing multiple helpful functions including digestion by processing carbohydrates and proteins through fermentation.

Digestion is like a processing station turning raw materials into energy to fuel the human body. Amazingly, the physiology textbooks have not yet caught up. In school, we grew up learning about digestion of protein, fats, and carbohydrates -- remember? Image 3 illustrates the anatomy of digestion as I review the basics for you.

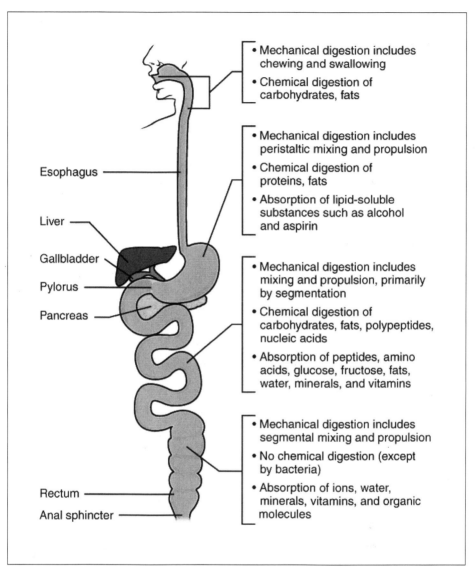

Esophagus

Liver

Gallbladder

Pylorus

Pancreas

Rectum

Anal sphincter

- Mechanical digestion includes chewing and swallowing
- Chemical digestion of carbohydrates, fats

- Mechanical digestion includes peristaltic mixing and propulsion
- Chemical digestion of proteins, fats
- Absorption of lipid-soluble substances such as alcohol and aspirin

- Mechanical digestion includes mixing and propulsion, primarily by segmentation
- Chemical digestion of carbohydrates, fats, polypeptides, nucleic acids
- Absorption of peptides, amino acids, glucose, fructose, fats, water, minerals, and vitamins

- Mechanical digestion includes segmental mixing and propulsion
- No chemical digestion (except by bacteria)
- Absorption of ions, water, minerals, vitamins, and organic molecules

Image 3: Mechanical and Chemical Digestion

Courtesy of OpenText: https://opentextbc.ca/anatomyandphysiology/chap-ter/23-7-chemical-digestion-and-absorption-a-closer-look/:

License: CC by: Attribution

The digestion of carbohydrates begins in the mouth by the action of ptyalin secreted by the parotid glands, which breaks down starches. This breakdown continues in the stomach where the food is joined by gastric secretions. The pancreas secretes the enzyme amylase into the duodenum, the first part of the small intestine. Within 30 minutes of the food and liquid called chyme reaching the duodenum, nearly all the starches have been converted to maltose and other small glucose polymers.

The cells on the villi of the small intestine contain the enzymes *lactase, sucrase, maltase,* and *a-dextrinase,* which split the polymers of glucose into monosaccharides such as glucose and fructose. These water-soluble monosaccharides are absorbed immediately into the bloodstream. That's why sugary foods leave us wanting more.

The digestion of protein takes a little longer. The stomach breaks protein into its constituent amino acids by the action of pepsin in a necessarily acidic environment (pH 2.0 to 3.0) precisely maintained by hydrochloric acid. When protein reaches the small intestine, the pancreas assists digestion with enzymes such as *trypsin, chymotrypsin, carboxypolypeptidase,* and *proelastase.*

The final stage occurs in the small intestine where the villi produce additional enzymes to split large polypeptides into tripeptides, dipeptides, and a few amino acids. These are then transported into the villi where the tri- and di-peptides all become amino acids and pass through to the blood.

Fat digestion is the slowest of all and helps us feel satiated. Fats are digested almost entirely in the small intestine first through emulsification by the action of bile, a non-enzyme liver secretion. Bile contains bile salts and lecithin, with lecithin attracting both water and fat. Mechanical mixing by peristalsis aids in the emulsification.

Pancreatic lipase then assists with the digestion of triglycerides to split them into free fatty acids and monoglycerides. The bile salts help transport the monoglycerides and fatty acids into the brush borders of the epithelial cells of the small intestine where they are absorbed into the blood.[40]

---

40   Guyton A, Hall J. (2016) *Textbook of medical physiology.* Philadelphia: Elsevier

This basic story has been around for the last 100 years but nowhere is there mention of microbes. In fact, the gut is like the largest factory you can envision with trillions of microbic employees working around the clock. For the last thirty years, we have known that microbes play an essential role in digestion of proteins and carbohydrates. But even now, the online encyclopedias mention the only role of bacteria in digestion as producing biotin and vitamin K.[41]

What we've learned in the last couple of decades includes this: Gram positive bacteria such as *lactobacilli* and *streptococci* inhabit the stomach at the level of $10^3/g$ and increase 1000-fold for a few hours after eating. At the junction between the small intestine and the large intestine, the microbial cell counts increase up to $10^{11}/g$.

To put these numbers, $10^3/g$ and $10^{11}/g$ in perspective, a gram (g) is approximately $1/4^{th}$ of a teaspoon which would hold about 5,000 grains of sugar. The number 10^3 is $10x10x10=1,000$. So, for $10^3/g$ if you visualize $1/4^{th}$ of a teaspoon of sugar, there would be 1 bacterium for every five grains of sugar. But with $10^{11}/g$ there would be 200 million bacteria for every grain of sugar! Amazing to wrap your mind around that, right?

By the time food reaches the large intestines, the transit time decreases considerably, so large colonies of bacterial communities develop and can reach $10^{12}/g$, some transient and some permanent.[42] Not to slight the enzymes and motion of the intestines, but think of the impact on digestion to have those huge, really immense numbers of bacteria working to degrade protein, carbs, and fats.

We now know that microbes in the large intestine contribute greatly to metabolism of food by producing hydrolytic enzymes, *butyrate, propionate,* and *acetate.* The process of fermentation uses these enzymes to digest 1) the remaining carbohydrates into short-chain fatty acids (SCFA), 2) proteins into

41   Digestion. https://en.wikipedia.org/wiki/Digestion Retrieved on 5-1-18

42   Macfarlane G, Macfarlane S. (2012) Bacteria, colonic fermentation, and gastrointestinal health. *J AOAC International* 95(1):50-60. https://doi.org/10.5740/jaoacint.SGE_Macfarlane

SCFA, branched chain fatty acids, and gas, and 3) undesirable metabolites that were not digested in the upper GI tract.

Lactate is also produced to regenerate cofactors needed in digestion. In addition, colonic microbes degrade and digest pancreatic secretions and mucins from the host.[43] WOW! Who could have predicted that microbes would play such diverse and important roles inside us? The truth is stranger than fiction; and we're still discovering.

· · · · · ·

L isten to this: our bodies even ferment small amounts of alcohol as a matter of digestive course all the time. This happens as carbohydrates and sugars are digested into SCFAs and proteins into their respective components. During this process, budding or true yeasts produce scant amounts of alcohol.

Over 35 years ago, Dr. N.I. McNeil of the London Medical School recognized the contribution of large intestinal fermentation to human energy intake,[44] but nutritionists have largely ignored this process to date, apparently deeming it insignificant. All branches of healthcare seem to have their scotomas, don't they?

Typically, the alcohol levels are barely noticeable in an otherwise healthy person. But this internal origin of alcohol known as "endogenous ethanol" is one of the major spots to understand how loss of homeostasis in the gut can cause ABS.

Blood alcohol levels are rarely studied in sober people because we tend to assume the level will be zero unless someone is drinking. Saudi Arabia has a zero tolerance for alcohol, so this study I'm about to summarize must really mess with their minds, if not their legal system.

---

43   Zihler A, Gagnon M, Chassard C, Lacroix C. (2011) Protective effect of probiotics on *salmonella* infectivity assessed with combined *in vitro* gut fermentation-cellular models. *BMC Microbiology* 11:264. http://www.biomedcentral.com/1471-2180/11/264

44   McNeil N. (1984) The contribution of the large intestine to energy supplies in man. *American Journal of Clinical Nutrition* 39:338-42

Researchers in Saudi Arabia measured endogenous alcohol in 1557 people of both sexes and thirteen nationalities. While the authors found no statistical significance for sex or nationality, it is interesting to note that the maximum value of BAC was 3.52 mg/dL or 0.00352%.[45] The median BAC value for all clusters was 0.04 mg/dL or 0.00004% - and NOT zero as would be expected for people who didn't drink any alcohol.

The production of endogenous ethanol (EnEth) in humans is not in question, only the amount. It seems most of what we normally produce is used as energy, but even then, tiny amounts of EnEth remain.

To summarize, the more acidic proximal colon ferments carbohydrate and produces short chain fatty acids (SCFA); The colon absorbs carbohydrates as they move along to the more alkaline pH of the distal colon where protein fermentation dominates. Protein fermentation generally produces scant amounts of ammonia (NH_3), hydrogen sulfide (H_2S), and other phenols generally thought to be detrimental to health.

Only carbohydrates are believed to produce endogenous ethanol, or alcohol. We all have minimal amounts of EnEth, but certain adverse health conditions such as renal failure and ABS can produce larger amounts. This is where we need doctors to recognize that yes, our bodies all produce small amounts of alcohol during the process of digestion; and some people, whose guts are out of balance with an overgrowth of yeast, can produce dangerously large amounts.

---

45   Al-Awahdi A. Wasfi I, Reyami F, Al-Hatali Z. (2004) Autobrewing revisted: Endogenous concentrations of blood ethanol in residents of the United Arab Emirates. *Sci & Justice* 44:149-152

CHAPTER 3 ~

PATIENT ZERO: JOE (PATIENT) AND BARBARA (JOE'S WIFE)

I have not touched a drink in a year
My blood alcohol levels seem queer
See my belly's a beast
It contains brewer's yeast
Any grains I eat turn into: beer

— *Phillip Gotica: Limerick Challenge (npr.org)[46]*

Barbara: *We're in the Emergency Room and I feel sick even though Joe is the patient. We've been here before, having him treated for alcohol poisoning and no one believing us that he hasn't been drinking. This is all so surreal.*

The lights are bright, and everyone is busy except for me -- I can only wring my hands and try not to let my stress over this thing trigger health problems of my own. This time Joe's blood alcohol level is 371mg/dL or .37% which is at least four times the legal limit in Texas (.08) and considered a near lethal emergency.

The ER doctor on call tonight is a jerk and tells me it's impossible for someone to be this drunk without drinking so Joe must be a closet drinker. When I challenge him, he explains that Everclear does not have odor and he must be hiding whatever he is drinking. He adds that many alcoholics are really good at hiding their drinking.

---

46   National Public Radio (2013) Limmerick Challenge. https://www.npr.org/templates/story/story. php?storyId=224547051 Retrieved July 21, 2018

I try with utmost patience to explain to him that I'm a nurse and I've been keeping very detailed records of Joe's condition. We use a Breathalyzer to track his breath alcohol concentrations (BAC) and that often he is drunk after having chewed gum with alcohol sugar or having eaten a chocolate-covered cherry that has liqueur in it. This doctor has his look of derision down amazingly well, and he uses it, as he again tells me "that's impossible."

In order to realize how devastating this is for both of us, you would have to know the kind of man Joe is: he's a steadfast, gentle, and loving man. He's one of the finest nurses I know; not just kind and compassionate, but someone who relates to patients, goes out of his way to comfort family members, and always educates patients about their illness and care.

We rarely go into a local store without running into a former patient or family member who stops Joe and thanks him for his care while they were in the hospital. Joe is the definition of responsible and dependable; he's never late to work, rarely calls in sick, and often stays over if he's needed to help during busy shift changes.

Joe and I met at the Veterans Medical Center in Salt Lake City through a mutual friend. Joe was working on the Neurology floor and I was working in Cardiac Critical Care. After a year of working together, Joe signed up for my Critical Care class and transferred to Surgical Critical Care where he took care of heart transplant patients.

We became good friends; often skiing or bicycling together on our days off, talking about his current girlfriend or my current boyfriend over lunch. It was ten years before our first date but when we finally kissed, I knew I'd been in love with him since the day we met.

······

The first time I remember an episode, some six years earlier, we were at my sister's house for Thanksgiving. Joe started acting very sleepy, was slurring his words and seemed extremely uncoordinated. He sat down in a chair, went to sleep and started snoring – and we hadn't even eaten dinner yet.

Family members asked me what was wrong with him and I said I had no idea. They were asking if he had been drinking or if he could be allergic to something he ate. I thought maybe he had low blood sugar. After about an hour, Joe woke up, ate dinner with us and seemed fine. We mostly forgot about the incident until six months later.

It was a Saturday in May. The weather was grand, and Joe and I had been physically working hard out in the yard most of the day. Around 3:00 in the afternoon we sat on the patio together and each of us had one beer, then showered and dressed. We had plans to drive to a nearby town for dinner and a movie.

Joe was driving, but when we got about 30 minutes down the highway, I noticed he was driving well above the speed limit and was weaving over the centerline. I asked him what was wrong, and I'll never forget the look on his face, because he turned his face to me, taking his eyes completely off the road, like he wasn't even driving. His eyes were foggy and red, his jaw was slack, his skin was bright red, and he slurred the words, "I'm fine," in such a drunken voice, I was terrified.

I started yelling at him to slow down, slow down, and all he could say was "I'm fine," in that same soggy voice. I screamed for him to "PULL OVER, PULL OVER Joe, because I need to drive!" Fortunately, Joe is an easy-going guy and he eventually pulled over and handed me the keys, but when I saw him try to walk to the other side of the car, I was alarmed. He bumped into the car, stumbled over his feet, and could barely open the door and get in without falling.

I drove the next 20 minutes to the restaurant and immediately asked them for some bread while we waited for a table. Once we got bread into Joe, he seemed somewhat better and I began to think he had an attack of severe hypoglycemia (low blood sugar). I talked to Joe about going to the doctor soon to get tested.

The next day I asked when he would go to the doctor, but he had no recollection whatsoever about the driving incident. He remembered nothing about speeding or weaving, or my yelling at him to pull over. I was shocked but was even more convinced it was hypoglycemia since diabetics in severe hypo- or hyper-glycemic states often act 'drunk' and may not remember their episodes. After this terrifying experience, the episodes started getting worse and closer together. As the episodes became more frequent, they began to blur together and overlap in my mind -- except for the hospital visits.

••••••

*T*he first time I took Joe to the ER, I thought he'd had a stroke. We'd been together all evening and he'd had two beers earlier in the evening but a couple of hours later, I heard him fumbling in the bathroom and I found him leaning against the wall urinating on the floor! I helped him to a chair and when I asked him what was wrong, he couldn't form even one word to answer me.

I called an ambulance and followed them to the ER, certain I would hear bad news about a stroke or perhaps his blood sugar. But instead, when we arrived, I was told his blood sugar was normal but his blood alcohol level (BAC) was a whopping 280mg/dL or .28%.

The legal limit for driving drunk in Texas is .08, so you can imagine my shock at hearing a number over three times that level. I was stunned and felt weak in my knees. The idea that Joe might have hidden and drunk an entire bottle of booze was incomprehensible. But I couldn't figure out what was happening; I began to ponder the previous episodes and realize that he indeed seemed drunk.

The doctors, who happened to be friends of ours, were kind during that hospitalization but I could see the disbelief in their eyes when I told them he'd only had two beers as they treated him for alcohol poisoning. He was admitted overnight with IV fluids and observation and released in the morning with a referral for counseling and AA. Joe and I were mortified that word would get around and all his colleagues would then think he was an alcoholic. My feelings of judgment, shame, and stigma were excoriating.

Of course, like so many family members would and do, I checked everywhere for alcohol. Even though I believed him, I didn't want to be in denial for what might really have been secret drinking. I marked our bottles of liquor and when the levels didn't change, I smelled and tasted them to see if they had been diluted. I checked the house, the garage, and Joe's truck to see if he was hiding bottles.

I even checked the finances and bank accounts to see if money was unaccounted for. I couldn't find any evidence anywhere that Joe was drinking more than I saw him drink. If he seemed drunk and admitted to two beers, I checked the garbage to ensure there were only two empty bottles there.

Often, he seemed excessively intoxicated after only two beers, which had never hap-
pened before this all started — two beers never used to faze him. Now, two beers sent him
to bed, where he was difficult to rouse. I used to worry that if the house caught on fire, I
wouldn't be able to wake him up to escape.

His snoring on those nights was horrendous. I tried to encourage him to go to a
doctor and at least get a sleep study for sleep apnea. But he looked at me in disbelief. Many
mornings he couldn't remember anything about the night before when he skipped dinner, or
we had an argument, or he went to bed early and passed out.

Joe: *In the beginning, I remember disorientation, euphoria; feeling drunk and not*
knowing why. Part of my brain was calm, but the other part was in a panic, not knowing
what was going on. There were mornings when Barb reminded me of events I didn't remem-
ber, and I thought 'Holy shit, I really don't remember that!'

I was in denial; I thought it wouldn't happen again, that it was an isolated incident.

Very early [circa 2003] *I thought maybe I had a tryptophan sensitivity because I*
always seemed woozy when I ate turkey, so I stayed away from turkey.

In summer 2004 I had a seizure while we were on a diving trip in Cozumel,
Mexico. The doctors ended up telling me it wasn't dive-related and that the seizure was
most likely caused by hyperthermia. But when I got back home, I had a complete workup
just to make sure: neurological, cardiac ultrasound, even a tilt table [to rule out causes
of syncope/fainting]. *All tests were negative, so I just kept on believing my other epi-*
sodes were food-related.

I remember falling off the porch at the Easter lunch at our pastor's house after
church and being driven home — I just thought I drank too much of whatever we were all
drinking. I was embarrassed because everyone from church was there. My pastor's now
grown children, Emily and Callie, still remind me how shocked and concerned they were
because it was so unlike me. Now that we can laugh about all this, they also lovingly call
me "Texas Jesus" for turning bread to beer.

B arb kept complaining about my snoring and telling me to get a sleep study done but I didn't believe I had sleep apnea. Besides, I already had a neurological and cardiac work-up and the doctors told me there was nothing wrong with me.

Often, I felt out of sorts at work, but I pushed through it. Co-workers would ask "what's going on? Do you need to eat?" They would check my blood sugar and it was usually low, so we all assumed I had hypoglycemia. They kept feeding me and I gained a lot of weight.

Somewhere in there, Barb talked me into doing my screening colonoscopy and I was diagnosed with high blood pressure; the doc put me on Bystolic and I really started having wild blood sugar swings. Sometimes it was 50, so everyone kept watching out for me and feeding me during episodes. I never thought I had high alcohol levels until later when I got taken to the ER a few times. But then I thought 'what the hell is that from?'

Barbara: *After the first ER visit, we purchased a Texas Department of Transportation (TxDOT) approved breathalyzer and began to record Joe's alcohol levels when he had episodes. I kept notes of what he ate prior to an episode, although often he didn't remember by the time I noticed he was drunk.*

Even now, it's hard for me to say the word "drunk" because the word is associated with excess drinking and I usually knew he'd had none or very little to drink. I witnessed it repeatedly: he'd be fine, and then, wham, it would hit him out of the blue.

Sometimes I would test his BAC – have him blow the breathalyzer – when he seemed fine, just to see what it was. Often his BAC would be 0.12 or 0.16% and he would seem perfectly okay. By the time he seemed drunk to me, his BAC would be .36% or sometimes even .40% and he would still be functioning when most other people would be unconscious with those levels.

I continually searched the literature for "alcohol sensitivity," "unexplained intoxication," anything I could think of to explain this absurd condition. Meanwhile the symptoms got worse and the episodes became more frequent.

Still at a loss, we conducted an experiment one night. Our adult son was visiting and Joe and I and our son and a friend all sat down together and blew the breathalyzer. We were all 0.00 as would be expected without any alcohol. We each chose a drink of beer (12 oz.) or wine (4 oz.) and visited as we drank our respective drinks.

Thirty minutes after finishing our drinks we each blew the breathalyzer. The two women at the table blew 0.04 and 0.03%. Our son tested at 0.02 and Joe blew a whopping 0.14%. What could possibly explain such a result? What would cause someone to be so sensitive to one drink of alcohol?

••••••

I can't tell you how many nights I prayed that Joe would be safe, and his drunkenness wouldn't come on while he was driving. I lived in fear of an accident where he or someone else would be injured. I was always the designated driver when we were together, but I couldn't drive him to and from work.

I told his friends to drive when they were with him and explained his problem as low blood sugar since I didn't know what else to say. Often eating did seem to help him, especially if I gave him a protein, like cheese – his worst episodes happened when he skipped a meal as he often did.

One winter night when I was driving home from work, I was planning to stop at the grocery store. But I heard a voice inside, telling me I needed to go straight home. When I pulled in the driveway, I knew something was wrong because it was getting dark, Joe was not in the house, and the door to the boathouse was open.

I ran down the backyard to the edge of the lake and saw Joe standing in chest deep water at the bulkhead looking very confused. He told me he couldn't figure out how to get out. The air temperature was 18° F. and the water temperature was around 40-45°. I ran to get a ladder, put it in against the bulkhead and mercifully, Joe was still able to climb the ladder.

He was getting hypothermic but still shivering, so I quickly got him out of his clothes and into a warm shower. He did remember the cold lake the next morning but had no memory of how he fell or what he was doing in the boathouse to begin with.

The trauma of dealing with a husband with an unknown condition was taking its toll. The concern for his safety was always in the back of my mind and I spent much of my free time searching for answers. I was at my wit's end. Sometimes he would pass out and I would worry he would stop breathing. I would debate about calling the ambulance, but I knew what would happen at the hospital — more disbelief from the doctors, treatment, discharge, and another big bill.

One morning in 2010 after church, we went to lunch and then stopped at a store. We'd been in the store about 30 minutes and I looked at Joe and could tell he was having an episode. By now they were happening very often and suddenly. He would get very pale and glassy-eyed and go to a state of "falling down" within minutes.

I asked a store employee to help me walk Joe to the car, which he kindly did. I remember asking Joe to give me the keys to his truck and he took them out of his pocket and tried to hand them to the store employee. I laughed to keep from crying.

Even though I usually took him home to go to bed, by now I was so frustrated that I thought maybe this time someone would listen to me. So, I drove him to the Emergency room where his BAC was tested at 0.378%. They started an IV and transferred him to the Intensive Care Unit (ICU). Again, the looks of pity from some, scorn and derision from others.

My dear friend and deacon, Susan Rushing, visited us in the ICU; later that night, she called me because she had hit on the term "Auto-Brewery" while searching the Internet. After that, I focused on the term Auto-Brewery Syndrome (ABS) and conducted search after search through my local college's library. I found very few articles, but at least it was there: this monster in our life had a name.

Joe: *The day Barb drove me to the ER and they sent me up to ICU, I was pissed off at the world. I couldn't believe there was something wrong with me. When I was told my BAC, I felt ashamed; I was shocked and humiliated. I thought it must be a mistake because I didn't have anything to drink but I knew people would judge me anyway. I remember threatening to check out AMA* [against medical advice] *but Barb reminded me that our insurance would not pay if I did that.*

After that hospitalization, Barbara strongly encouraged me [I think he first said, 'hounded the crap out of me' and then changed it] *and the lightbulb went on - where I realized I needed to see someone. I knew Dr. McCarthy from working at the hospital and since he is a Gastro guy, I agreed to go.*

In retrospect, I remembered I had been given antibiotics after I broke my foot and had surgery; Ancef 1Gm; erythromycin p.o. for three weeks. That was about the time this all started.

Barbara: *Dr. McCarthy was a godsend! When Joe and I first went to him, I could tell he was skeptical, but I could also feel the scientist in him was intrigued. He took the articles I had copied for him, read them and proceeded to do a complete GI workup and treat Joe the way the case studies recommended.*

Joe was one of the fortunate ones: he was diagnosed with ABS with the underlying yeast of S. cerevisiae, treated with medication, a low carb diet, and probiotics and responded immediately. Work made him test his BrAC before every case and he always blew .00 after that.

He maintains a moderately low carbohydrate diet, abstains completely from alcohol, and has been symptom free for over eight years. Both Joe and I will be forever grateful to Dr. Justin McCarthy for listening to us with an open mind. In one way, he's a hero; but in another way, he's the epitome of what all diagnosticians should be – a physician-scientist with compassion. Thank you, Justin!

CHAPTER 4 ✐

METABOLISM OF ALCOHOL

There is more wisdom in your body than in your deepest philosophy.

— *Frederick Nietzche*

People have fermented alcoholic beverages for millennia and alcohol (technically ethanol or ethyl alcohol) is ubiquitous in American culture. We treasure alcohol; it influences our subconscious perception of events, improving our experience of food, music, and socializing. It lowers inhibitions and charges personal events in a way that makes us want to repeat them. In moderation, alcohol ignites our senses, helps us relax, and provides our hearts with some positive benefits.[47]

We often consider alcohol harmless but drinking alcohol can be beneficial or dangerous depending on your age, health status, intake amount, and timing. When we drink, the alcoholic beverage permeates all the tissues in the body nearly immediately, from the stomach to the circulatory system and into the brain. For this reason, we measure alcohol levels in the bloodstream.

Blood alcohol concentration (BAC) for medical purposes in the United States is typically measured in milligrams per deciliter (mg/dL). Detection ranges from a lower limit of 10 mg/dL to 400 mg/dL considered potentially lethal. A BAC of 400 mg/dL translates to .40% of your blood being alcohol meaning four drops of every 1,000 drops of blood is pure alcohol!

Breath alcohol concentrations (BrAC) are usually calculated in milligrams percent (mg%). So, a BAC of 80mg/dL would translate to a BrAC of

---

47   National Institutes of Health. Rethinking Drinking. https://pubs.niaaa.nih.gov/publications/ RethinkingDrinking/Rethinking_Drinking.pdf Retrieved: 10-31-18

.08% which by the way, is the legal limit currently in all states.[48] The mg% is the more common usage in the U.S. so healthcare providers might tell someone with a BAC of 40mg/dL that their level is 0.04%. In daily conversation, we drop the % and just say .04. Don't get confused though. Remember to look for the units of measurement, especially if you are in Canada or the U.K. since labs there use other units of measurement such as mg/L.

Image 4 shows the levels of impairment of alcohol at various Blood Alcohol Concentrations (BAC). These levels are important not only for law enforcement but also for medical treatment of intoxication.

---

48   Dalawari P. (2014) Ethanol Level. https://emedicine.medscape.com/article/2090019-overview

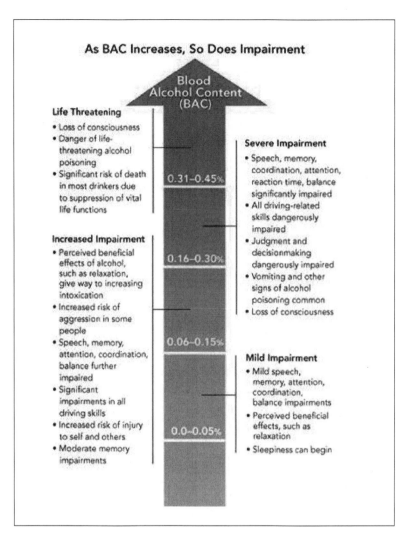

Image 4: Levels of Impairment of Alcohol Correlated to BAC

https://pubs.niaaa.nih.gov/publications/AlcoholOverdoseFactsheet/Overdosefact.htm

License: CC: by Attribution.

Each U.S. state regulates alcohol laws and as mentioned all states set the legal limit for intoxication at 0.08% with varying penalties. Some states charge a person driving at this alcohol level with a Driving While Intoxicated (DWI) and other states use the term Driving Under the Influence (DUI) or even Operating Vehicle while Intoxicated (OVI). The Federal Government, through the Federal Motor Carrier Safety Association, sets the legal alcohol limit for all commercial drivers at 0.04%.[49]

Alcohol is a central nervous system depressant and the body responds to it as it would a controlled substance or poison. I probably don't have to tell anyone that it can be detrimental to health, even at low levels. Fortunately, adult bodies are resilient, and have mechanisms in place to detoxify alcohol. However, some of the remaining by-products of alcohol detox, such as acetaldehyde, are toxic to our tissues and take longer to detoxify and be eliminated.

DETOXIFICATION

To understand ABS, we must understand the process of alcohol detoxification to look for clues and connections. While yeast is the main culprit of the gut dysbiosis, there may be other errors in processing alcohol that contribute to ABS.

When drinking, ethanol diffuses from the stomach capillaries into the nearby major liver cells where some of the ethanol is detoxified by enzymes to inactive products. This process is called metabolism, and the products are called metabolites depicted in Image 5. The enzymes help speed up metabolism, but the amount, type and speed of the enzymes can vary from person to person.

---

49   Federal Motor Carrier Safety Association. What if I Fail or Refuse a test? https://www.fmcsa.dot. gov/regulations/drug-alcohol-testing/what-if-i-fail-or-refuse-test. Retrieved: 10-31-18

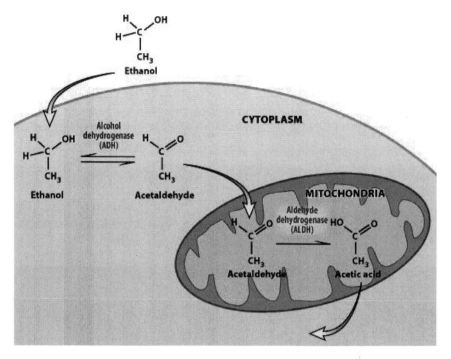

Image 5: Metabolism of Alcohol in the body:

Image courtesy of RD Schwartz-Bloom, Duke University

STAGE 1 OF ALCOHOL METABOLISM: ETHANOL TO ACETALDEHYDE

While some alcohol is metabolized in the stomach, the primary site of metabolism is in the liver. The liver is a meaty, half-moon organ on the upper right-side of your abdomen that filters toxins and produces an array of life sustaining chemicals and enzymes. Take care of your liver because you cannot live without it.

One liver enzyme, alcohol dehydrogenase (ADH), along with a liver coenzyme, catalyze the oxidation of ethanol to acetaldehyde.[50] Typically, we have enough ADH to metabolize the alcohol in one drink within an hour or

---

50   Sarcola T, Iles M, Kohlenberg-Mueller K, Eriksson C. (2002) Ethanol, acetaldehyde, acetate, and lactate levels after alcohol intake in white men and women. *Alcoholism* 26(2):239-245

so and that rate remains constant. We metabolize most alcohol with the liver enzymes, but we eliminate about 5-10% unchanged in the breath and urine.

We can see that the ADH molecules will become overwhelmed if the rate of drinking increases more than one per hour. That's when alcohol accumulates in the bloodstream and leads to more severe intoxication which alters mood and behavior, and can damage the brain, heart, and other organs. Another obvious danger associated with episodic inebriation is injuries. Alcohol is a factor in about 60% of fatal burn injuries, drownings, and homicides, 50% of severe trauma injuries and sexual assaults, and 40% of fatal motor vehicle crashes, suicides, and fatal falls.[51]

Drinking during pregnancy can cause disabilities to the baby known as Fetal Alcohol Spectrum Disorders (FASD). According to the National Institute on Alcohol Abuse and Alcoholism, "There is no known safe amount of alcohol – even beer or wine – that is safe for a woman to drink at any stage of pregnancy."[52]

STAGE 2 OF ALCOHOL METABOLISM: ACETALDEHYDE TO ACETIC ACID:

Another liver enzyme, acetaldehyde dehydrogenase (ALDH) along with a substance called glutathione, goes to work metabolizing acetaldehyde into an inactive compound called acetate. Eventually, acetate is converted into carbon dioxide and water, and sometimes isopropanol in our cells.[53]

Here comes the veisalgia, better known as a hangover: the body's ability to produce ALDH can be overpowered by excessive drinking, which then allows acetaldehyde to build up. Remember the intermediary alcohol metabolite, acetaldehyde, because many of us in the ABS community believe it to be a big piece of the puzzle and I will discuss it later in relation to symptoms.

51   National Institutes of Health. Ibid

52   Alcohol's Effects on the Body. https://www.niaaa.nih.gov/alcohol-health/alcohols-effects-body Retrieved: 10-31-18

53   Dwyer J, Tamama K. (2013) Ketoacidosis and trace amounts of isopropanol in a chronic alcoholic patient. *Clinica Chimica Acta* 415:245-249. https://doi.org/10.1016/j.cca.2012.10.057

Acetaldehyde is where the pain of alcohol metabolism comes in because it is relatively toxic to humans and leads to the nausea, headache, and lethargy of a hangover. Leafy green vegetables can help rid our bodies of acetaldehyde by inducing more ALDH, but really, who wants to eat veggies when you are hungover?

METABOLIC ABNORMALITIES

Strangely, some people lack the ability to metabolize acetaldehyde quickly and completely with ALDH. They may experience the facial flushing, headaches, nausea, vomiting, and rapid heart rate like a hangover when drinking even small amounts.[54] But interestingly, this genetic variation may provide a protective effect for alcoholism by repelling the drinker long before addiction can set in.

There is quite a bit of information on a variation of the ALDH enzyme in Japanese and Han Chinese people that makes them more sensitive to the effects of alcohol.[55] Many Asians have a mutation of the ALDH2*2 gene that decreases the enzyme production and thus reduces alcohol tolerance in about one-third to half of the population. Most people with low tolerance, choose not to drink.

Many in our ABS support group wonder if our patients have this or some other genetic alteration or enzyme deficiency. So far, I have not found a connection between ABS and the genetic variation of ALDH, but I don't believe anyone has looked for it. Even though over thirty ABS cases were reported in East Asians in the 1970s,[56] no mention was made of a link between ABS and the genetic variation of ALDH in Asians. We believe there may be another closely related or similar genetic link for ABS.

---

54 Gender Matters: How is alcohol eliminated from the body? https://sites.duke.edu/apep/module-1-gender-matters/content/content-how-is-alcohol-eliminated-from-the-body/. Retrieved: 2-14-18

55 Ushida Y, Talalay P. (2013) Sulforaphane accelerates acetaldehyde metabolism by inducing aldehyde dehydrogenases: Relevance to ethanol intolerance. *Alcohol & Alcoholism* 48(5):526-534

56 Kaji H, Asunuma Y, Yahara O, et al. (1984) Intragastrointestinal Gut Fermentation Syndrome: Report of Two Cases and Review of Literature. *J Foren Sci Soc* 24(5):461-471

We haven't seen a racial connection either, but genetics might be a fruitful avenue of ABS research. Nearly all the 250+ patients I have been in contact with are Caucasian males, including a dozen or so from other countries (England, Australia, Canada, Germany and the Czech Republic) but genetic profiles keep showing us how small our world really is and there may be another connection.

We all recognize that people react differently to different drugs, and alcohol is no exception. Biochemists Bernard Testa and Stefanie Kramer tell us that many biological factors influence the metabolism of foreign compounds such as alcohol, including inter-individual factors (written in the genome) and intra-individual factors (which change over time). The metabolic reactions are "so many, so varied, and of such immense importance… that they represent at present an apparently unsurmountable challenge to entirely successful predictions of drug metabolism."[57]

The ABS support group also ponders the possible link of ABS to the metabolism of medications and toxins like acetaldehyde. We think there may be a physiological error somewhere in either processing alcohol or in ALDH production (see Appendix A) that may or may not be genetic. Perhaps a genetic mutation link, or race or ethnicity link will be discovered in the future, but right now the literature is mute on the subject.

ALCOHOL ABSORPTION FROM OTHER ROUTES

Physiology and medical textbooks do not discuss absorption of alcohol from any other avenue except the stomach because it is not well-known or researched. However, one study shows that rubbing alcohol is absorbed through our skin in amounts detectable in the bloodstream when applied for cooling purposes or from hand sanitizers.[58]

---

57   Testa B, Kramer S. (2009). The biochemistry of drug metabolism – an introduction. Part 5: Metabolism and bioactivity. *Chem Biodivers* DOI: 10.1002/cbdv.200900022

58   Rosano T, Lin J. (2008) Ethyl glucuronide excretion in humans following oral administration of and dermal exposure to ethanol. *J Analyt Toxico.* 32(8):594-600

The practice of alcohol enemas is even more interesting for our purposes of studying ABS. According to Columbia University's *Go Ask Alice* health questions website,[59] the practice of putting alcohol into the rectum causes more rapid absorption than drinking and thus a quicker buzz. But the risks are real and serious – so please don't try it!

Alcohol enemas are very dangerous because excessive alcohol levels are reached quickly and the body's survival mechanism of vomiting excessive alcohol from the stomach is bypassed. Plus, there are several reports of severe colitis and death after alcohol enemas.[60,61]

This practice is not new. According to the National Institutes of Health, there is evidence on ancient pottery that Mayan people practiced enemas ritualistically using alcohol and other intoxicating substances in order to reach ecstatic states.[62]

I only mention this practice here because in ABS alcohol is produced in the intestines, either small or large depending on where the yeast has colonized. These experiments by daring and foolish people are showing us something important about the physiology of having alcohol bypass the stomach – that intoxication occurs more quickly and produces a far more intense effect. Our patients can testify to this effect.

While I certainly want people to abstain from the practice of alcohol enemas, researchers might be able to gain insights about alcohol metabolism and ABS by studying this risky business. And for the record, many of our patients would dispute that the vomiting mechanism is bypassed because they quite frequently experience nausea and vomiting when flaring!

---

59   Alcohol Enemas. Go Ask Alice at Columbia University: Health Questions. https://goaskalice. columbia.edu/answered-questions/alcohol-enemas

60   HuffPost: Butt Chugging Leads To Severe Alcohol Poisoning Of University of Tennessee Student. (2012) https://www.huffingtonpost.com/2012/09/25/butt-chugging-wine-alcohol-enema-university-of-tennessee-pi-kappa-alpha_n_1913575.html

61   Wilson Jackie. (2012) Experts: Alcohol Enemas Extremely Dangerous. https://www.cnn. com/2012/09/26/health/alcohol-enemas/index.html. Retrieved 11-5-18

62   National Institutes of Health. A multidisciplinary approach to ritual enema scenes on ancient Maya pottery. https://www.ncbi.nlm.nih.gov/pubmed/3528674 Retrieved: 8-27-18

DRUNKY MONKEY

An interesting side note is that humans aren't the only animals to have an impulse for alcoholic fermentations; apparently several species like to get drunk as well. Scientists have documented ten or more animals such as bats and monkeys that get high on intoxicating plants.[63]

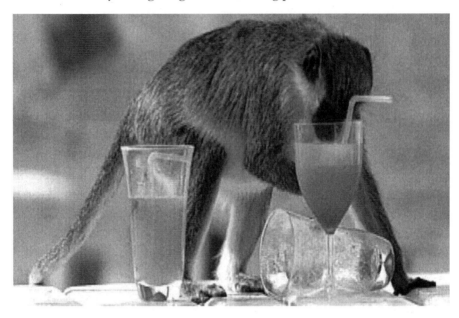

Image 6: Monkey Drinking

Courtesy of: John Downer Productions (Weird Nature for BBC)

Vervet monkeys on the island of St. Kitts used to eat fermented sugar cane but now have adapted to sneaking cocktails from tourists in the area. Most monkeys drink in moderation but much like humans, about 12% drink heavily, 5% drink excessively, a small tribe abstain completely, and juveniles drink more than adult monkeys.

---

63   Muller N. (2011) Animals Getting High: 10 Common Drunks. http://www.australiangeographic. com.au/topics/wildlife/2011/10/animals-getting-high-10-common-drunks/

Bats, on the other hand, don't seem to metabolize alcohol the way we do even though they eat fermenting fruit with up to 4.5% alcohol. Biologists discovered bats in Belize can use their sonar without ill effects even with blood alcohol contents that would be well over the legal limit for humans. Maybe someday we'll even discover other species that auto-brew.

······

In humans, chronic alcohol ingestion is dangerous. Persistent alcohol use, or in the case of ABS, alcohol exposure, can create health issues with the heart such as cardiomyopathy, the pancreas such as pancreatitis, and the liver such as cirrhosis. It also puts the person at higher risk of certain cancers such as head and neck, liver, colorectal, and breast cancers.

Chronic alcohol exposure increases the risk of sleep disorders, depression, stroke, immune suppression, bleeding from the stomach or esophagus, problems managing diabetes, high blood pressure, and weight, and sexually transmitted infections from unsafe sex. Other long-term consequences of alcohol include psychological or behavioral changes and unfortunately, chronic addiction.

ABS patients have all these risks from their endogenous alcohol, and to fully understand ABS, we must look at the biological, medical, and cultural impacts of alcohol exposure and even alcoholism.

CHAPTER 5 ～

DIPSOMANIA

Four Horsemen-Terror, Bewilderment, Frustration, and Despair

— *Alcoholics Anonymous*

Don't you think the things people are most ashamed of are things they can't help?

— *C.S. Lewis, Till We Have Faces*

Imagine you're in the throes of Auto-Brewery Syndrome but you're being treated like an alcoholic. And worse, you're being treated like it's your fault; as if there's something to be ashamed of; as if you are in denial, and if only you had enough will power you could get well.

In nursing school, I learned to withhold judgment. I learned that alcoholism, like mental illness, is a disease; that people don't choose to have a disease. Yet, every time I took Joe to an Emergency Department (ED), at least a few of the providers, mostly MDs, treated us with antipathy; we felt like scum.

There's a term in EDs, "frequent flyer" to describe someone who shows up in the ED quite often. Many times, frequent fliers are in pain and have chronic health issues that are difficult to treat. Sadly, the term has become code for someone with drug-seeking behavior or mental problems. I didn't want to become a frequent flyer in the hospital where we both worked, so I stopped taking Joe to the ED. To think he could have died because I was afraid of what the doctors would think of us!

Suppose Joe was an alcoholic rather than having ABS during those visits; where is the compassion? I know ED docs are trained to implement extraordinary life-saving measures after trauma – and they do; but even if they believe the trauma is self-inflicted, as in drinking, why wouldn't they remember that alcoholism is a disease, treat us kindly, and make a compassionate referral?

••••••

Alcohol use disorder, colloquially known as alcoholism, is a serious public health crisis that affects between 12 and 13% of Americans. Alcoholism is on the rise with 23% of people under 30 years of age meeting the medical criteria. Unfortunately, societal attitudes about moral choice and free will still override our knowledge of the disease model and we continue to stigmatize addicted patients and their families.

Many experts agree with research psychiatrist Dr. Nora Volkow, Director of the National Institute on Drug Abuse, that addiction is a disease of the brain, but society and healthcare still treat addiction as if it has to do with willpower.[64] Dr. Volkow says she is certain that social environments, developmental stages, and genetics are intimately linked to the vulnerability to addiction and recovery, but neuroscience continues to add knowledge to the brain disease model of addiction.

Dr. John Fortney and co-researchers in Little Rock, Arkansas conducted a study on 733 at-risk drinkers and examined the perceived public stigma for alcohol use and treatment.[65] The subjects reported substantial levels of perceived stigma for alcohol use (86.1%) and judgment by members of the community for their seeking primary care treatment for alcohol use disorders (48.9%).

64   Volkow N, Koob G, McLellan A. (2016) Neurobiologic advances from the brain disease model of addiction. *N Engl J Med* 374:363-371 DOI: 10.1056/NEJMra1511480

65   Fortney J, Mukherjee S, Curran G. et al. (2004) *J Behav Health Serv & Res* 31: 418 https://doi.org/10.1007/BF02287693

More importantly, subjects reported perceived stigma from their primary care providers because they were at risk drinkers (35.7%). Respondents also reported a consequential lack of privacy with primary care treatment (42%).

Nurses Justin Sleeper and Dr. Shelley Bochain conducted research on the *Stigmatization by Nurses as Perceived by Substance Abuse Patients.*[66] Patients voiced common themes of feeling that staff placed their own needs above those of the clients which decreased the clients' comfort and increased their anger and frustration.

People who feel judged or undervalued tend to avoid seeking care and in general, have poorer outcomes. Just like when I stopped taking Joe to the ED because of the stigma. We might have found treatment sooner if I had kept taking him and demanding answers.

••••••

ABS is a hellish ordeal, like getting tangled in a fence of concertina wire: patients first get inebriated for no clear reason, then often suffer a huge hangover. They must then untangle themselves to figure out what's going on and sometimes experience days of recovery from alcohol poisoning only to get snagged and scratched again and again.

But the lingering wound is addiction. Sadly, because patients with ABS are exposed to alcohol in extremely high levels and often daily for years, they can become habituated to the effects of alcohol and begin to crave it. First, let's step back and look at alcohol addiction in general.

How could someone get addicted to alcohol if the after-effects of drinking are so repellant? Well, addiction happens both physically and psychologically and those aspects are intertwined in what we refer to as the body-mind connection. When the body is physically addicted, it's not simply a question of mind over matter anymore. We see how little control we have over our actions when our bodies are hijacked by a poison.

---

66   Sleeper J, Bochain S. (2013) Stigmatization by nurses as perceived by substance abusing patients: A phenomenological study. *J of Nurs Educ and Pract* 3(7):92-98. http://dx.doi.org/10.5430/jnep.v3n7p92

Dipsomania is an antiquated word used for alcoholism and derives from the root "dipsa" meaning thirst, and "mania" meaning excessive enthusiasm. I doubt any alcoholic would tell you they are enthusiastic or thirsty, but cravings often commandeer their behavior. One member of AA told me: "Alcoholism is when the desire for alcohol becomes a compulsion and that's all you think about. It's an allergy of the body combined with a malady of the mind."

To look at the psychological aspect of addiction, we turn to Dr. Hitoshi Morikawa in *The Journal of Neuroscience*, who said a key distinction in understanding addiction is that alcoholics are not addicted to the experience of pleasure or relief they get from drinking alcohol. They are addicted to the "experience of the moment" including the environmental, behavioral and physiological cues.[67] These feelings are reinforced when alcohol triggers the release of dopamine in the brain.

"People commonly think of dopamine as a happy transmitter, or a pleasure transmitter, but more accurately it's a learning transmitter," said Morikawa. "It strengthens those synapses that are active when dopamine is released." Alcohol, in this model, is the enabler. It circumvents the dopaminergic system and tells our brain that what we are doing at that moment is rewarding and thus worth repeating.

It's a profound irony that people with ABS are often wrongly accused of being a closet alcoholic, but then due to lack of effective diagnosis and treatment become addicted to alcohol. We first need to research effective diagnosis and treatment for ABS and then must educate the medical community on the syndrome and the ramifications of its sequelae.

Most importantly, we need to continue working on shifting the culture within the medical community to stop shaming patients. Reproach, humiliation, blame and shame have no place in healthcare. We must embrace the disease model to find compassion for those with ABS, addiction from ABS, and for all people with addictions.

---

67   Nauert R. (2015) Subconscious Memory and The Lure of Alcohol. *Psych Central.* https://psychcentral.com/news/2011/04/13/subconscious-memory-and-the-lure-of-alcohol/25271.html Retrieved: 11-6-18

CHAPTER 6

AN ONGOING NIGHTMARE: NICK (PATIENT) AND KAREN (NICK'S WIFE)

The world breaks everyone and afterward many are strong at the broken places.

--Ernest Hemingway

Nick's story is one of the hardest one for me to narrate because he is still suffering from GI symptoms, setbacks and ABS relapses. He is one of several ABS members in our support group whose illness appears to be chronic rather than acute. He seems to have other GI conditions working against his ABS. My heart breaks for Nick and the other patients who continue to suffer without relief.

Nick's symptoms of nausea, vomiting, and abdominal pain started in 2011 when he was 30 years old. He had been to numerous doctors in Ohio who could not discover a diagnosis for all his gastro-intestinal manifestations. Nick's wife Karen contacted me in September of 2013.

Karen: *For the past two years, my husband wakes up every morning and vomits. This is accompanied by severe abdominal pain. At times, he will behave as if he were intoxicated, though he hasn't had a drop to drink. He's had endoscopies, colonoscopies, gastric emptying tests, HIDA (hepatobiliary), MRI and CT scans which all show that structurally his GI system is functioning as it should; however, he continues to suffer from strong acid reflux, with belching and vomiting after some meals.*

The specialists are stumped. Can you recommend tests to help diagnose auto-brewery or leaky gut syndrome? Any additional information you can provide would be greatly appreciated.

Karen was one of the first caregivers to contact me after I published the case study on Joe, and I felt an immediate kinship with her. Like me, Karen had been searching the Internet to find out what could possibly be causing Nick's health issues and found me through a CNN news article on the case study. She felt that Joe's story of ABS answered so many of their questions and when they bought a breathalyzer and got high readings, all of Nick's symptoms made sense.

Their primary doctor referred Nick to a holistic doctor in early 2014. When Karen showed him the news article about my case study, he acknowledged he had only heard of ABS but was willing to talk to me and learn what I knew. I realized then he must be an exceptional doctor.

Karen: *When I first told Nick about ABS, he didn't think he was drunk - why would he be drunk when he didn't have anything to drink?! The new doctor was the first to diagnose ABS and try and treat what was going on with his gut. He ordered a test that showed 4x the normal yeast level in his system. The doctor put him on a diet and had him journaling; we really focused on him getting a lot of rest too. Nick wanted to try healing without medication if he could.*

At that point Nick lost his job and was in school, so we just made sure he stuck to a consistent sleep schedule, which is hard when you're sick; this really does take a toll - with your circadian rhythms too; he can't always sleep just because it's dark.

At that time, I was completely overwhelmed, so my mother, who lives in Hawaii, said, "Why don't I take him for a couple of months and follow the plan of care to make sure he eats what he's supposed to eat while he's here." When he came back, it was a complete 180; he had followed the diet and was like a different man; so much better.

Within a month, however, he slowly started to get occasional flare ups, and I just dismissed it; I thought, 'Oh, maybe it just happens on occasion – I'll take that over it happening every day'. But it progressively got worse. That's when my mom said, "Send him

back again; you can't be dealing with this, trying to work, and start a family," and so he
returned to my mom's house.

From June 2014 to April 2015 I received numerous requests for inter-
views and many of the radio and TV shows also wanted to have a patient
tell their story. Nick and Karen were very open about Nick's diagnosis and
agreed to every interview and TV show that called.

I also formed a professional bond with their holistic doctor, Dr. Anup
Kanodia, who trained at Harvard. A holistic M.D., Dr. Kanodia already knew
a lot about yeast infections but he reached out to me to learn more about
ABS. He also was willing to be interviewed for the TV shows and the four
of us appeared in episodes of 20/20, BBC, and "World's Weirdest Events"
among others (see links in the Introduction).

Karen had a business meeting in San Antonio, TX in the fall of 2014
and Nick was going with her. Joe and I drove to San Antonio just to meet
them because we had grown so close to each other through emails and phone
conversations. Both Joe and Nick admitted it was good to know someone else
with ABS who could relate to the horrific disease. Nick was not quite cured
of ABS since he was still having occasional episodes or flares but talking to
Joe who had been symptom-free for four years seemed to give him hope.
Unfortunately, his hope was short lived.

3-5-15: Karen: *I was wondering, Nick is almost back to square one again so it's
another month in Hawaii possibly followed by the Diflucan – are you aware of any ongoing
or proposed research on this? There need to be more studies to convince the naysayers. I am
thinking of contacting the CDC, American Gastroenterological Association, maybe some
other universities, since Nick has offered to be a case study and be placed under observation.*

For the next 18 months Nick continued to struggle with his health and
have appointments with Dr. Kanodia. Nick preferred holistic approaches
over medication, but he finally took two rounds of fluconazole and nystatin
with only short-term relief. His symptoms abated when he went to Hawaii
where he could focus on his health and diet, but he would relapse when he
returned to Ohio. Karen and I discussed the possibility of environmental

exposures in their home and she and Nick had their home tested. The results came back negative.

9-9-16: Karen: *I can't tell you how many people have approached us with severe stomach problems, not necessarily auto-brewery, but they have no diagnosis or treatment. I have to believe there is a correlation somewhere between antibiotics, the food we eat, stress, etc. and the gut. Last time I visited our Gastro department at the medical center, the waiting room was jam packed! Nick has been on three rounds of antibiotics because of awful kidney stones the past 5-6 weeks. I'm hoping it doesn't undo all the progress with his auto-brewery. I will keep you posted.*

2-11-17: Nick to the support group: *I just wanted to post in support of ALL the loved ones and spouses of the people with ABS... my wife Karen has been THE ONLY reason I'm still alive today and without the support of someone who truly cares, this condition can get out of hand quickly, ending up with someone in jail or a mental health facility...*

If you haven't already, please look into Dr. Anup Kanodia and Dr. Barbara Cordell's research and if you need to, find the videos we made in hopes to educate people and bring awareness to this truly terrible condition.

I am ALWAYS free if anyone wants to inbox me to chat in private to discuss the other perspective of this condition... as someone who has suffered with this for 6-7 years, I can try to give the best feedback possible :).

As far as the spouse perspective, which I BELIEVE is the worst side of this disorder, you can contact my wife Karen and I'm SURE she will do her best to help in any way...I believe, me handling this illness, and being sick almost daily is WAY easier than what I've put my wife through ALL these years and what she has endured.

Most importantly, I hope EVERYONE stays in a positive mindset and I believe with us all sticking together and supporting one another, we can do what we can to relieve the stress of feeling alone through these rough times.

2-12-17: Nick (in response to posted question): *I have not had a major toll to my liver or kidneys although that has been a big worry for me. I'm constantly having* general blood draws to determine my kidney and liver function, to keep a close eye on them; but am lucky to say they are doing fine.

8-2018: Karen: *We're seeing, yet again, another specialist. Nick's still not well. His ABS and vomiting symptoms are not all day long like they used to be; I don't know what the difference is and the few times he goes to Hawaii, it kind of seems like it knocks it back a little bit more. It's less severe and then over time it gets worse and worse and worse again. So, we found that sending him to Hawaii about once a year really helps. I know that stress and sleep is a huge component of it, so I think he gets an opportunity to really rest up and get a lot of sun and fresh air. And the trigger still may be the home we live in. He stayed away from the house a couple of weeks without relief so maybe he needs to stay out a month or two.*

We saw a new gastroenterologist; a brand new one, because the last one we saw said Nick is a closet drinker and that I needed to look around the house. So I finally got approval for the insurance and the new doctor was great, but after the last endoscopy, he said the chair of the department doesn't recognize this illness (Auto Brewery Syndrome) and so he would treat it as gastroparesis. I said 'this is what you guys did six years ago and it didn't do anything. I don't understand why you can't work with these doctors in New York who have cured one gentleman and at least see what they've learned.' But they don't even want to reach out to them!

We are now connected with a holistic center and we are taking a different tactic; we see an FNP [Family Nurse Practitioner]. We don't want to see a doctor and I've found the best luck with nurse practitioners. We're going into this without telling them the diagnosis — just the symptoms and they want to do blood tests and stool samples and we'll see what they recommend based on that. This FNP's focus is the microbiome.

When we go to the GI doctors, the GI waiting areas are always full; and you can't tell me there isn't a correlation between our diet, toxins, stress, and GI problems.

Nick has ADHD; so, staying on top of him to follow the regimen is like babysitting and I have to check up on him. But I don't know if ABS is exacerbated by his ADHD. He's not on medication right now for ADHD. He is on Wellbutrin. He had a bad depressive episode a few months back; he was just not himself.

His boss called me – (Nick works 2-3 days a week when he can handle it). Fortunately, his employer is understanding and accommodating when Nick has a flare up. His doctors do have him on Wellbutrin now and they talked about ADHD meds but he's wary of any medication.

Nick and I are going to try acupuncture for his nausea. He hasn't been able to keep food down very well. It's really, really bad; it's worse in the morning – he will vomit; sometimes water won't even stay down. I have to force him to drink Pedialyte or an electrolyte drink. He's been flaring about 8 months now with daily vomiting. His mid-section looks like a beer gut – like that beer gut kind of guy – and that's what he has: bloating, and some fat.

He's on the daily probiotics, but you have to figure out what to take, and we've never found out what's missing from his gut so hopefully this NP will know what to recommend. There are so many claims for cures, you could go mad to try everything out there.

I think our health is only going to get worse; with all the crap they've allowed us to consume and that goes in our food; this is only the tip of the iceberg and 10-20 years from now we're going to see major issues with our microbiome and immunity.

I thought maybe there was an environmental component, or lack of Vitamin D so we upped his Vit D recently to see if that would help. He's on probiotics and a multivitamin. What's so odd, is that when he gets really, really bad, the only food he can seem to stomach is Chipotle. I don't know if it's just because – well it's high carb but he manages to keep it down. It's so weird. I wonder if he's going into detox and feels miserable, so he eats carbs?

He goes through waves and cycles: when he's down, he's done with it – and the depression is too real; he really just wants to just end it all. He figures if he were dead, he wouldn't suffer anymore.

I hope the NP has some good recommendations. I'm hoping acupuncture will work for his nausea. He is open to it, but asking someone with ADHD to sit still with needles in him?

POSTSCRIPT

Nick is still flaring from time to time. Karen and Nick keep pushing the envelope for treatment options from conventional to integrative. They are still on a roller coaster of emotions from hope to despair and back to hope. Nick continues to manage symptoms through lifestyle adjustments. This is when our healthcare system seems the most broken to me; when we cannot find answers to such a debilitating set of symptoms. Maybe he has several other conditions in addition to his diagnosed ABS, but no one has been able to find them. I pray Nick can wake up from his nightmare soon.

CHAPTER 7 ⌒

THE ASTONISHING HUMAN MICROBIOME

Messieurs, c'est les microbes qui auront le dernier mot.
(Gentlemen, it is the microbes who will have the last word.)

— *Louis Pasteur*

If you haven't yet read much about the human microbiome - the sum of all the microbes (bacteria, archaea, fungi, and viruses) living in and on our bodies - prepare to have your mind blown – and grossed out a little. I've been a science nerd since I was very young, and I got hooked on human physiology in high school. I was learning a new language and loved words like borborygmi for the gurgling sounds made by our stomachs, epistaxis for a nosebleed, and xerostomia for dry mouth.

Through nursing school and beyond, it became my hobby to read the latest discoveries about our amazing and complex bodies. My study of physiology includes microbiology but our knowledge about the trillions of microbes living mostly in harmony on our bodies is new within the last couple of decades. Scientists have barely scratched the surface and even then, it has been mind-boggling to try and keep up with the research.

THE TREE OF LIFE

In order to better understand the microbiome, a short review of the Tree of Life is in order. The tree of life is a metaphor used as a visual tool to explore life and the relationship of organisms to one another.

In the early 20ᵗʰ century, scientists divided all life into "animal" and "plant" but by the 1950s, that system of classification was suddenly inadequate because it failed to include bacteria, fungi, and protists. At that point, Thomas Whittaker classified life into five Kingdoms: 1) Bacteria and Actinobacteria (which are Prokaryotes previously known as Monera), 2) Plants, 3) Animals, 4) Protists and 5) Fungi (the last four of which are Eukaryotes).[68]

Prokaryotes are single-celled organisms lacking a nucleus and membrane-bound organelles. Eukaryotes are organisms consisting of a cell or cells with a nucleus in which the genetic material is DNA in the form of chromosomes.

In the 1970s, microbiologist Carl Woese found a new kink in the Tree, that prokaryotes can be divided into two distinct lineages, or lines of descent as well: bacteria and archaea. Today, we consider these divisions to form two out of only three domains of life with the third being all the eukaryotes.[69] Image 7 shows a representation of the currently accepted, three-pronged Tree of Life.

68   Annenberg Learner. Evolution and Phylogenetics: A Brief History of Classification. https://www.learner.org/courses/biology/textbook/compev/compev_2.html Retrieved: 11-8-18

69   Prokaryotic cells. https://www.khanacademy.org/science/high-school-biology/hs-cells/hs-prokaryotes-and-eukaryotes/a/prokaryotic-cells Retrieved 11-8-18

Phylogenetic Tree of Life

 = You are here

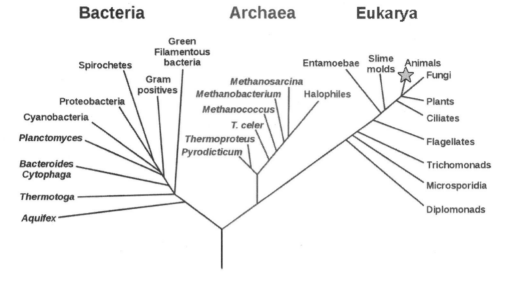

Image 7. Current Tree of Life

Courtesy of: OpenStax CNX. Located at: http://cnx.org/contents/185cbf87-c72e-48f5-b5le-fl4f2lb5eabd@l0.8. License: CC: by Attribution.
(credit: a modification of work by Eric Gaba)

These three divisions are then broken down into phyla (shown on the tree) and then to several other classifications and finally genus and species. Remember learning in high school biology that humans are called *homo sapiens?* This is the Latin genus and species labeling and we use a specific genus and species (and sometimes sub-species) for every living organism identified so far.

Viruses are typically not included on the Tree of Life for many reasons which are hotly debated; they don't share characteristics with celled life, they donate and steal genetic material, and they require a host to live. Stay tuned for more science on that topic. But of course, that's not the only debate.

In his recent book, *The Tangled Tree: A Radical New History of Life,* David Quammen details how scientists have genetic evidence that the branches on the tree of life are not so distinct from one another as we currently think.[70] Organisms from different branches can, and often do, transfer genes 'horizontally' to each other in addition to 'vertically' from parent to offspring.

Horizontal gene transfer explains why bacteria acquire resistance to antibiotics so quickly; they can transfer antibiotic resistant genes back and forth among species the way we send each other text messages.

This information tells us that family and species lineages may be very intertwined and may be changing, or evolving, much more quickly than we realize. Even the Tree of Life shows us just how wonky and dynamic science can be. I'll be interested to see the new tangled tree develop (sorry, Darwin).

••••••

The preeminent text of human physiology for over fifty years is Arthur Guyton's best-selling *Textbook of Medical Physiology.*[71] I've always kept a current copy on my bookshelf. However, the 2000 edition barely mentions bacteria in the gut (exactly five sentences), let alone the microbiome. Guyton's contribution at the turn of the 21st century includes:

> Numerous bacteria, especially colon bacilli, are present even normally in the absorbing colon. They are capable of digesting small amounts of cellulose, in this way providing a few calories of extra nutrition to the body…Other substances formed as a result of bacterial activity are vitamin K, vitamin B12, thiamin, riboflavin, and various gases that contribute to *flatus* in the colon, especially carbon dioxide, hydrogen gas, and methane. (p. 763)

In the section on "Composition of the Feces," Guyton goes on to say that 30% of the feces is made up of *dead bacteria* and the products of bacteria cause the odor depending on a person's "flora" and the type of food they eat.

70   Quammen, D., (2018). *The tangled tree: A radical new history of life.* New York: Simon & Schuster

71   Guyton A. Hall, J. (2000) *Textbook of Medical Physiology.* St. Louis: Elsevier

"Flora" denotes "plants" in botany and is not technically correct when applied to the human gut microbiome. If Dr. Guyton came back to life today, he would likely be stunned to see the vast number of studies and astounding science on the human and gut microbiome.

Thankfully, textbooks that specialize on gastroenterology are finally, if only barely, starting to talk about the role of the microbiome. A 2009 gastroenterology textbook dedicated exactly 10 of its 3442 pages to the microbiome in the section of "Basic Mechanisms of Normal and Abnormal Gastrointestinal Function" under the heading "Miscellaneous."[72]

The textbook summarizes the science on the microbiome and how much there is yet to learn, but with no mention of Gut Fermentation Syndrome or even fermentation in the gut as a normal part of digestion. Here's another scotoma - unreal.

So, ask your GI doctor if he or she did a residency before or after 2009? It's no wonder that doctors look at us with blank stares when we claim to have Auto-Brewery Syndrome – even the information on the microbiome is not in the medical school curricula yet and barely in continuing education.

MORE MICROBE THAN HUMAN

Conceptualize this: the number of human cells in our body is currently estimated at 30 trillion (3.0×10^{13}). We also host a whopping 1.3 to 2.3 times more microbial cells or genes in or on our body than we have human cells.[73] That means *more of our DNA is microbial than human*. Seriously, re-read that sentence, and let it sink in.

For 25 years scientists estimated the ratio of bacterial to human cells at 10:1. Based on new science, they revised the estimates in 2017 of the ratio to the 1.3 to 2.3:1 but it still seems fair to say that we are more microbial than human.

---

72   Ley R, Gordon J. The human intestinal microbiota and microbiome in Tadataka, Y., and Alpers, D., (2009) *Textbook of Gastroenterology* (5th Ed.) West Sussex: Wiley-Blackwell: 635-644

73   Sender M, Fuchs S, Milo R. (2016) Revised estimates for the number of human and bacterial cells in the body. *PLoS Biol* 14(8): e1002533. https://doi.org/10.1371/journal.pbio.1002533

The definition of the human genetic microbiome is the entire collection of genes found in all the microbes associated with a particular host.[74] This includes the skin, mouth, nasal passages, alimentary canal (from mouth to anus), lungs, and the urogenital system (bladder, urethra, and for women, vagina, cervix, and uterus), each with its own characteristic microbiota.

When the human genome was completely sequenced in 2003, we discovered we have 25,000 genes.[75] This may sound like a lot until you realize the simple fruit fly (*Drosophila melanogaster*) has 17,000 genes, the Norway spruce (*Picea Abies*) has 28,384 genes, and the common Poplar tree has 45,000 genes!

Furthermore, scientists hypothesize the microbiome plays a greater role in health and illness than our genes. These perspectives on the microbial and human DNA ratios and relationships elicit the core philosophical and spiritual question of what it means to be human, right?

••••••

The non-human microbes in and on us include bacteria, fungi including yeasts, and archaea. Bacteria are single-celled microorganisms that contain cell walls but not a nucleus and have their own branch on the Tree of Life. I'll discuss shortly how bacteria help us maintain life and health.

Fungi are unicellular, multicellular, or syncytial spore-producing organisms feeding on organic matter. Remember, they are part of the Eukaryote branch of life between plants and animals. The fungus branch includes molds, yeasts, mushrooms, and toadstools.

We're really drilling down here to arrive at the cause of ABS because yeasts make up only 1% of the Fungal Kingdom. Most yeasts reproduce by fission or dividing in two; but the true yeasts reproduce by budding or producing a bleb or daughter cell, from the parent. Most of the yeasts found in ABS are from the class of budding yeasts in the family *Saccharomycetaceae*. This

---

74   Shugart E, Lontok A. (2016) Which microbe are you? Human Microbiome Edition. Washington, DC: American Academy of Microbiology. https://www.asm.org/Browse-By-Audience/Higher-Education-Educator#k12 Retrieved: 7-6-19

75   All about the human genome project: https://www.genome.gov/10001772/ Retrieved: 6-24-18

is the same family of the genus and species *S. Cereviseae* used to make wine and beer. Godisgoode, remember?

Archaea are single-celled microorganisms with no nucleus but with distinct molecular differences from bacteria. Because they live in unbelievably extreme environments, archaea are also known as "extremophiles".

One example is the critters thriving in the up to 235° F. geysers and vents in Yellowstone National Park called, and I am not kidding, *Nitrosocaldus yellowstonii*.[76] Another example is *Picrophilus*, isolated in soil in Japan that is the most acid-tolerant organism known; capable of growth at around an incredible pH 0! Extreme, right?

The extremophiles we all know though are the methanogens, which as their name suggests, produce methane gas; thus the stench found in cattle yards, some odors seeping from the ground from marshes and hot springs, and part of the stink of human gas[77] (yes, farts).

These preposterous organisms, once thought to live only in the most inhospitable places, also reside inside us. Archaea were discovered in the human gut over 20 years ago but have largely been ignored because they don't cause problems as far as we know. However, we may discover someday that some of these miniscule cells impact health and illness.

······

Babies in the womb live and grow in a sterile environment, so where do we get all our microbes? Well, we start by gathering them in the birth canal. As a mother gives birth, she is coating her infant with vaginal fluids teeming with microbes. This means the mother is inoculating her baby moving through the birth canal, with her microbiome.

Babies born by caesarean section will still be able to collect microbes from the environment, but they are not receiving the microbe-rich bath from mom. The microbiomes of C-section babies end up being quite different

---

76   Kan J, Clingenpeel S, Macur R, et al. (2011) Archaea in Yellowstone Lake. *ISME Journal* 5:1784-95

77   Niederberger T. Archaea. https://www.britannica.com/science/archaea Retrieved: 6-15-18

from naturally born babies and researchers are beginning to discover the implication of these differences on health later in life.

For several generations we thought we were doing women a favor by surgically removing the baby, but microbes are one huge reason this is simply not a good practice. You pregnant moms should know that a C-section can save lives but should only be used in an emergency.

Breast-fed babies also glean microbes and amass their microbiomes from their mothers' milk. The initial thick colostrum is like baby's second vaccine – supercharged with immune components. Mom's milk is dynamic, custom-made, and changes as her baby grows. Breastmilk can change from day to night and even respond with additional antibodies when her baby is sick based on a message from the baby's saliva. Amazing, isn't it? Science has never been able to even replicate mothers' milk, let alone improve on it.

Bottle-fed babies will still acquire a set of microbes from their formula plus the environment, but their microbiomes will be very different from those of breast-fed babies. These differences last a lifetime and scientists are just starting to research the ramifications of those differences.

The establishment of our microbiome starts like a window box, clean and empty. The initial soil and compost, or microbes are added through birthing and feeding as well as touching the environment. The gardeners, or family and friends participate in adding soils and nutrients or microbes, but the garden, or baby has a say as to what it accepts. Our genes largely pre-determine the remainder of our microbiomes by genetic selection which occurs through chemical communication as well as temperature and moisture levels; amazing.

······

But Houston, we have a problem! We know the microbiome plays a huge role in life itself, but the current technology has yet to catch up. Microbiology laboratories can only culture about 1% of the microbes in the human gut by conventional microbiology procedures. The most common technique uses shallow, sterile plates with a medium such as agar in them. Technicians inoculate the medium with the human tissue or fluid and place the plates in incubators for a certain amount of time. Once the time has elapsed, lab techs count the microbes under a microscope.

The number of cells from natural environments, such as our guts, that grow viable colonies on agar medium and can be counted by microscopy is very low for most organisms. James Staley and Allan Konopka coined the term "Great Plate Count Anomaly" in 1985 to describe this inability to culture gut bacteria *in vitro,* or outside the body.[78]

The most popular explanation of why microorganisms do not grow in isolation is that of mutualism; where some species require certain metabolites of other species and some marine species must be paired with others in order to grow.[79] In other words, I'll scratch your back, if you scratch mine.

An example of mutualism in the human gut is when bacteria breakdown proteins into component parts and in return, the bacteria receive a steady supply of food. But we don't know if this mutualism requires several species working together. And it's nearly impossible to determine which pairs have positive interactions among the trillions of microbes.

The Great Plate Anomaly means the vast majority of the microbes in our environment, on our bodies, and in our guts remain inaccessible for study. Finding the 99% of the missing diversity remains one of microbiology's greatest challenges.

Only recently have scientists begun to develop innovative techniques to study more of our microbes. Instead of culturing, scientists can now extract DNA and identify the microbial genomes but not all labs have the capability yet.

78   Staley J, Konopka A. (1985) Measurement of in situ activities of nonphotosynthetic microorganisms in aquatic and terrestrial habitats. *Ann Review Micro* 39:321-346. https://doi.org/10.1146/annurev.mi.39.100185.001541

79   Epstein S. (2013) The phenomenon of microbial uncultivability. *Cur Opin Micro* 16:636-642 https://doi.org/10.1016/j.mib.2013.08.003

Sierra, one of our support group members says, *"It is a laboratory cell culturing technique. You can't kill single-celled organisms and still identify them easily. These days genetic testing is done after a lab tech grows more of the living creatures in petri dishes. Glamorous job - keeping the poop creatures alive? As a professional scientist, I've done similar tasks, so I know the technique well. They grow them, identify them under microscopes and by genetic testing, and then they test various medicines on them to see what works to kill them."*

Over the last decade, many of the studies conducted on the gut microbiome have concentrated on identifying and cataloging bacterial species by 16S rRNA technologies. The simple identification and sequencing do not provide information regarding function. Nor has it included fungi and yeasts in the taxonomy of the microbiome until very recently.

·······

Fortunately, only about 1% of the trillions of bacteria in and on us causes disease -- and only then when our microbiome is disturbed and an organism, or two or three, can take hold and grow out of control. This is why several people in the home may get sick and not others.

Think of an invasive plant species like English Ivy. In its native habitat in England, Asia and Africa, English Ivy is considered a lovely ground cover or even a building decoration. But in the U.S. this plant is considered invasive in your lawn. The different soil and climate conditions are what allow the plant to over-grow viciously and invade your lawn.

Of course, an infection (whether bacterial, fungal, or viral) requires three factors: 1) the microbe or the opportunistic pathogen, 2) external environment or transmission, and 3) susceptibility of the host.

For example, if you get athlete's foot, caused by a fungus (the invasive seed), it's because something in your microbiome (the soil and climate) is out of balance that creates a vulnerability that enables the fungus to grow. The microbe is a fungus known as *tinea pedis*. The external environment, or transmission, may be someone with the fungus on his or her feet showering in the gym shower right before you; in our lawn analogy it would be a bird dropping those invasive seeds in your grass before the rain.

If your skin microbiome is in good defensive shape, that fungus won't have a toe hold (ha). However, you may be susceptible if your natural immune system is weakened – then the fungus can get a purchase and suddenly you wake up a few days later itching like crazy.

······

Normally the trillions of bacteria, viruses, fungi, and archaea residing in and on your body exist symbiotically with you and compete with potentially hazardous microbes to prevent opportunistic pathogens from encroaching. The recise word for species living together without injury is "commensal", or more accurately "eating together at the same table."

Commensal bacteria, and fungi can prevent microbes from colonizing on your skin by competing for nutrients, by secreting chemicals that repel the pathogen, or by stimulating the immune system to overcome the pathogen. *Malassezia furfur* and *Candida albicans* are examples of fungi, more accurately yeasts, found on the skin of humans.

Microscopic mites (eight-legged bugs) live on us too. We all have them, so no point in getting squeamish. *Demodex folliculorum*, found in hair follicles, and *Demodex brevis*, found in sebaceous glands, are examples of mites that are commensals. On occasion they over-colonize and cause disease, but again, only if the microbiome is in dysbiosis; meaning the good microbes are fewer than needed to keep the potential pathogens in check. Isn't the microscopic world fascinating?

Some of our commensals can even over-colonize if host conditions are in disequilibrium, and then will themselves cause health issues. For example, we all have *Staphylococcus aureus,* more commonly known as *staph* on our skin. *Staph* is a commensal gram-positive bacterium that can easily cause an infection if conditions are right.[80] The seeds are already there, but the soil has to change for it to overgrow.

Frighteningly, our microbiomes are shifting toward more pathogenic states. In a national U.S. study, the prevalence of *S. aureus* in nasal cavities decreased from 32.4% in 2001-2002 to 28.6% in 2003-2004. Unfortunately, the more hostile methicillin-resistant *S. aureus* (MRSA) increased from 0.8% to 1.5%.[81] As the less virulent staph goes down, the more pernicious variety goes up; something is happening to mutate our seeds and maybe change our soil too.

Now, of course, a typical microbiome might be vastly different for those living in one country versus another, or even from region to region. The microbiome is an incredibly dynamic system as we have seen, and we may have very different microbiomes depending on our age, location, community and season. These differences in our personal and collective ecosystems affect health and disease.[82,83]

The microbiome can vary according to factors such as gender, use of antibiotics, diet, and educational level, and can vary by body site.[84] Get this: your right hand shares just a sixth of its microbial species with your left hand. And within 24 hours of moving into a new dwelling we spread our own microbes around, turning the new place into a reflection of ourselves.[85] How unbelievable is that?

80   Oregon State University. (2013) Gut microbes closely linked to proper immune function, other health issues. *ScienceDaily* September 16 www.sciencedaily.com/releases/2013/09/130916122214.htm Retrieved: 6-20-18

81   Gorwitz R, Kruszon-Moran D, McAllister S, et al. (2008) Changes in the prevalence of nasal colonization with *S. aureus* in the United States, 2001-2004. *J Inf Dis* 197:1226 –34

82   Yatsunenko R, Rey F, Manary M, et al. (2012) Human gut microbiome viewed across age and geography. *Nature* 486:222-228. http://www.nature.com/nature/journal/v486/n7402/full/nature11053. html

83   Davenport E, Mizrahi-Man O, Michelini K, et al. (2014) Seasonal variation in human gut microbiome composition. *PLOS* 9(3):1-10. http://journals.plos.org/plosone/article?id=10.1371/ journal.pone.0090731

84   Ding T, Schloss P. (2014) Dynamics and associations of microbial community types across the human body. *Nature* 509: 357-367. http://www.nature.com/nature/journal/v509/n7500/full/ nature13178.html

85   Yong E. (2016) *I contain multitudes: The microbes within us and a grander view of life.* UK: Bodley Head

THE GLORIOUS GUT

The gut is like a vast and intricate hub of highways connected to every other city in the body by the circulatory system including the brain, the hormone system, the circulatory system, the hepatic and digestive systems, and the limbic system. We usually think of the intestines as the sewer of the body; a tube that rids all the other cities of waste and toxins. But it also serves as the nurturer through digestion and metabolism, and the protector by playing a major role in immunity. Perhaps we should think of the gut more as the central processing plant.

But in addition to the processing functions, the gut-brain connection is no joke. Have you ever had a "gut" feeling? Or experienced butterflies in your belly? And those butterflies can come from either stress nerves or excitement? The brain has a direct effect on the gut and vice versa!

The gut has even been dubbed the "second brain" because it plays a huge role in our feelings and emotions. The neurons in the intestinal lining and the vagus nerve are constantly transmitting to and receiving messages from the primary brain. The chemical mood regulators known as serotonins and endorphins are produced in both brain and gut and influence our mood and mental health.[86]

But that's not all. In addition to being part of the digestive, metabolic, and immune systems, the gut microbiome may even be a neglected organ of the endocrine system.[87] Diabetes is associated with loss of gut microbiota diversity and there is now a confirmed association between the gut and glucose metabolism disorders.[88]

Historically, we've studied digestion, immunity, mental well-being, metabolism and endocrine as separate functions, but we are finally seeing

---

86   Hadhazy A. (2010) Think twice: How the gut's "Second Brain" influences mood and well-being. *Scientific American* https://www.scientificamerican.com/article/gut-second-brain/

87   Clarke G, Stilling R, Kennedy P, et al. (2014) Gut microbiota: the neglected endocrine organ. *Mol Endocrin* 28:1221-38

88   Stefanaki C, Peppa M, Mastorakos G, Chrousos G. (2017) Examining the gut bacteriome, virome, and mycobiome in glucose metabolism disorders: Are we on the right track? *Metabolism* 73:52-66. http://dx.doi.org/10.1016/j.metabol.2017.04.014

the intimate, complex, and inseparable interactions between the microbiome and almost all other body systems. We need to de-partition these complex processes in order to better understand them.

All these marvelous functions of the gut have to do with the microbes inside us. And again, much of this information is only in the academic and science journals and has yet to make its way into the general college and medical textbooks. Plus, don't you think the gut needs a more glorious name and reputation?

••••••

My focus zooms in here to the gut microbiome to increase our understanding of Auto-Brewery Syndrome caused by fermentation which originates in the gut. Some of our doctors diagnosing ABS found the culprits in the proximal or distal large intestine while others cultured samples taken from various locations in the small intestine.

The gut microbiome is like our proverbial garden. If we only eat refined processed food, the rich soil may dry up and turn to dirt that will only allow weeds to thrive. If we add fresh organic nutrients which are like fertilizer for the soil. Then the soil of the microbiome becomes like compost, rich and able to sustain the processing functions like a well-tended garden. We can nurture the microbes in the soil to nourish the whole body, grow the proper defenders, and even bolster our mental health.

According to the American Academy of Microbiology, the intestines and colon contain one of the densest known microbial communities on Earth.[89] Our understanding of how diet affects gut microbes is still limited, but we know that dietary variation even between winter and summer can cause fluctuations in the composition of the intestinal microbiome.[90]

---

89 Shugart, Ibid.

90 Hullar M, Fu B. (2014) Diet, the gut microbiome, and epigenetics. *Cancer J* 20(3):170-174. http://journals.lww.com/journalppo/Abstract/2014/05000/ Diet,_the_Gut_Microbiome,_and_Epigenetics.2.aspx

Furthermore, we now know there are significant differences in gut microbes between people in different countries that are apparent in infancy as well as adulthood.[91] One study that reviewed metagenomes from nine countries in three continents assessed the distribution of gut subspecies and found several of the subspecies were geographically specific. For example, *Eubacterium rectale* was found almost exclusively in the samples from China.[92] These facts are just begging for more research.

••••••

Because our understanding is so new, we don't really even have a benchmark of what constitutes a "normal" gut microbiome. Don't give up yet, though. Through the groundbreaking scientific work of the American Gut Project, and other research studies, there is hope of discovering a baseline to answer questions like: What is a typical gut microbiome? How do "ours" compare to "others" depending on many of the factors mentioned above, such as age, gender, location, and diet? And most importantly, how can we improve our gut microbiomes?

According to their website, http://americangut.org/about/, "The American Gut Project, an Earth Microbiome Project study co-founded by Dr. Rob Knight and Dr. Jeff Leach, is the world's largest crowd-funded citizen science project in existence." Since 2012, the project has enabled regular people like you and me to submit stool samples for identification of microbes -yes, Joe and I have done it! Just think, you too can learn the composition of your poop and contribute to research. **#poopforscience**

Part of the money you pay to have your own microbes analyzed allows researchers to collect samples in developing countries and contributes to the scientific efforts to answer questions about associations between the microbiome in health and disease. So, come on, pay for your poop information as well as a good cause.

---

91   Ghosh T, Gupta S, Bhattacharya T, et al. (2014) Gut microbiomes of Indian children of varying nutritional status. *PLOS* 9(4) http://journals.plos.org/plosone/article?id=10.1371/journal.pone.0095547

92   Costea P, Coelho L, Sunagawa S, et al. (2017) Subspecies in the global human gut microbiome. *Molecular Systems Biology* 13:(960):1-11

The American Gut Project has sequenced 4,658 microbiota samples from 3,624 people, including 179 participants in the Personal Genome Project. According to preliminary data, "At the phylum taxonomic level, the major players are Firmicutes and Bacteroidetes".

Firmicutes include *Clostridium* and *Lactobacillus* species and many producers of the short-chain fatty acid butyrate. Butyrate provides many protective functions to the intestinal lining. Bacteroidetes includes *Bacteroides* and *Prevotella* genera, both of which break down polysaccharides.[93] This information could provide insight into sugar metabolism and weight management.

Another recent study explored relationships of archaea (those weird extremophiles) and fungi of the gut microbiome with diet and bacterial residents of the gut. The study examined 96 gut samples from volunteers who were free from chronic GI issues, diabetes, cardiac disease, and immunodeficiency syndromes. The scientists detected *significant correlations* of the yeast and fungus populations with different bacterial compositions as well as long term and recent dietary intake.[94]

From this and other research, we are beginning to understand that complexity and diversity of microbes in the gut may play an important role in a healthy gut.

······

In his book *Rewild*,[95] Jeff Leach describes his time with the Hadza people in Tanzania, where he lived for over a year. The Hadza are hunter-gatherers living much the way their ancestors survived for generations which puts them in contact with the natural microbial world. The people that Leach studied do not keep livestock or plant food at all, but instead forage for their food. Furthermore, they breast-feed their children for at least two years, have

93   Leach J. (2015) Preliminary characterization of the human gut population. http://humanfoodproject.com/preliminary-characterization-of-the-american-gut-population/

94   Hoffmann C, Dollive S, Grunberg S, et al. (2013) Archaea and fungi of the human gut microbiome: Correlations with diet and bacterial residents. *PLoS ONE* 8(6):e66019. https://doi.org/10.1371/journal.pone.0066019

95   Leach J. (2016) *Rewild*. San Bernardino, CA: Human Food Project

limited access to medicines such as antibiotics, drink untreated water, and occasionally eat uncooked meat.

Leach and his team conducted studies on the composition of the gut microbiomes as well as many other sites of microbes in, on, and around the Hadza people. He compared those results with samples from people with a more typical Western diet and found the Hadza to have a much more diverse set of microbes. After sharing the local diet for two weeks, Leach discovered his own gut microbiome had changed dramatically to be more in line with the Hadza.

The Hadza people not only have extraordinary diversity in their guts compared to Westerners, but also have a low number of *Bacteroides* and an astonishingly high number of *Prevotella* with dozens of species compared to only two in the West. Leach's conclusion is that Westerners have lost up to half of the diversity of their gut microbiome.

We don't yet know the implications of this loss, but looking at the rates of obesity, autoimmune disorders, and other "modern" plagues, we can surmise that loss of diversity may be contributing to our problems. It is possible that our overuse of antibiotics, the homogenization of staple crops, and the amount of processed food we eat are all shrinking the biodiversity of our collective and individual ecosystems.

The good news is, our bodies are resilient, and our guts can change in just a few weeks by reintroducing foods that help restore the soil in the garden, so to speak.

THE MICROBIAL AVENGERS

In addition to digestive, metabolic, and waste functions, some of our gut microbes are like superheroes playing a critical role in regulating immunity. Macrophages, produced in larger numbers in the gut than anywhere else in the body, are like Avengers that go out into the bloodstream to defeat many of the invading villains including viruses and even cancer.

For decades, we've been told our immune system has the amazing ability to distinguish between "self" and "non-self". So, you may be wondering by now how our immune system can still work when confronted with dozens of microbial species that are commensal and yet can suddenly transform into a pathogen. The early discoverers of the microbiome wondered the same thing.

A 2016 article in *Nature* on the microbiome and immunity pondered the science behind that exact conundrum.[96] The more complete picture of immunity is nothing short of stunning; there are intimate, inseparable, and keenly balanced interactions between immunity and metabolism, with the microbiome as the mediator. Scientists labeled this interaction "crosstalk." Of course, the crosstalk, or mutualism, occurs by an array of enzymes and chemical signals whereby our microbes interact with the innate immune system.

We actually have two immune systems: one is innate and the other is adaptive. The innate system consists of the skin and cellular barriers, inflammation, the complement (eliminating pathogens with antibodies), and natural killer cells. The adaptive immune system includes lymphocytes and passive and active immunity (think vaccines).

Among all the functions of the gut microbiome, from providing energy, to synthesizing vitamins and nutrients, to maintaining health, one of the most important is maintenance of the intestinal epithelium or lining, even while being exposed to a myriad of outside influences from food and drink to medicines and toxins. Without this barrier-like protection, our GI systems would become inflamed and inflammation is the basis for, or an accompanying factor in, nearly all diseases.

A disturbance in the gut microbiome can lead to immune dysregulation and eventually to autoimmune disorders.[97] When the immune system no longer recognizes its host, it can go rogue and begin to destroy tissues in

96   Thaiss C, Zmora N, Levy M, Elinav W. (2016) The microbiome and innate immunity. *Nature* 535:65-74. DOI: 10.1038/nature18847

97   Wu H, Wu E. (2012) The role of gut microbiota in immune homeostasis and autoimmunity. *Gut Microbes* 3(1):4-14. PMID: 22356853 DOI: 10.4161/gmic.19320

the body. The results are diseases like rheumatoid arthritis, multiple sclerosis, Type I diabetes, and psoriasis.

The organs of the immune system include the tonsils, thymus, bone marrow, spleen, and lymph nodes. A few physiology and medical texts include Peyer's patches, small clusters of lymph tissue throughout the ileum that prevent pathogenic bacteria from infecting the intestines. But current texts and graphics should really include the intestinal epithelium as well as the gut microbiome as integral parts of the immune system.

YEASTY BEASTIES

Only in the past few years have scientists begun to study the small but complex role of the fungal portion of the gut microbiome – the myco-biome. This may be the most important section of the science in our quest to understand ABS because the diagnosing doctors and researchers believe the mycobiome is the storm center. Commensal yeast turned pathogenic in the intestines ferment carbohydrates into ethanol.

We know the incidence of fungal-related infections is on the rise and is increasingly associated with chronic diseases such as cystic fibrosis. A 2016 article in *Current Fungal Infections Report* states that for years the focus of microbiology for cystic fibrosis (CF) was on *Pseudomonas aeruginosa*. But an increasing body of evidence points to the role of molds and yeasts contributing to the pathogenesis of CF.[98]

Fungi also play a role in inflammatory bowel disease and obesity. Dr. Irina Leonardi and her colleagues demonstrated that certain immune system phagocytes cruise around the intestines and bolster antifungal immunity. A genetic deletion of those specific phagocytes caused colitis-like symptoms in mice. Polymorphisms of those phagocytes were detected in patients with

---

98   Williams C, Ranjendran R, Ramage G. (2016) Pathogenesis of fungal infections in cystic fibrosis. *Curr Fungal Inf Report* (10):163-169. DOI: 10.1007/s12281-016-0268-z

Crohn disease and they were unable to produce antibodies against multiple fungal species.[99]

Dr. Mar Rodriguez and collaborators demonstrated that specific fungal compositions were associated with obese patients and could be further classified as "healthy" and "unhealthy" obesity. They showed that species of *Mucor racemosus* and *M. fuscus* predominate in non-obese subjects, but the abundance could be reversed by weight loss.[100] This information could be huge in developing innovative treatments to address obesity.

······

Immuno-compromised patients and neonates often contract opportunistic invasive fungal infections;[101,102,103,104,105,106] however, very little research has been done on yeast overgrowth in otherwise healthy subjects. I found one study with subjects who had symptoms of yeast with no definitive conventional diagnosis; symptoms included fatigue, headaches, poor concentration, GI distress, muscle pain, joint pain or urogenital symptoms.[107]

99   Leonardi I, Li X, Semon A, et al. (2018) CX3CR1+ mononuclear phagocytes control immunity to intestinal fungi. *Science* 359(6372):232-236. DOI:10.1126/science.aaol1503

100   Rodriguez M, Perez D, Chavez F. et al. (2016) Obesity changes the human mycobiome. *Scientific Reports* 5:14600. https://www.nature.com/articles/srep14600

101   Behbod B, Sordillo J, Hoffman E, et al. (2015) Asthma & allergy development: Contrasting influences of yeasts & other fungal exposures. *Clin Exp Allergy* 45(1):154–163. DOI:10.1111/cea.12401

102   Riquelme A, Calvo M, Guzman A, et al. (2003) *Saccharomyces cerevisiae* fungemia after *S. boulardii* treatment in immunocompromised patients. *J Clin Gastroenterology* 36(1): 41-43. http://journals.lww.com/jcge/Fulltext/2003/01000/Saccharomyces_cerevisiae_Fungemia_After.13.aspx

103   Olver W, James S, Lennard A, et al. (2002) Nosocomial transmission of *Saccharomyces cerevisiae* in bone marrow transplant patients. *J Hosp Inf* 52(4):268-272

104   Ascioglu S, Rex J, DePauw B, et al. (2002) Defining opportunistic invasive fungal infections in immunocompromised patients with cancer and hematopoietic stem cell transplants: An international consensus. *Clinical Infectious Diseases* 34:7-14. https://doi.org/10.1086/323335

105   Rimek D, Redetzke K, Kappe R. (2006) Impact of antifungal prophylaxis on the gastrointestinal yeast colonization in patients with haematological malignancies. *Mycoses* 49(Suppl 2):18-23. https://doi.org/10.1111/j.1439-0507.2006.01319.x

106   Parra-Herran C, Pelaez L, Sola J, et al. (2010) Intestinal candidiasis: An uncommon cause of necrotizing enterocolitis (NEC) in neonates. *Fetal Ped Path* 29:172-180. https://doi.org/10.3109/15513811003777342

107   Lewith, G., Chopra, S., Radcliffe, M., et al. (2007) Elevation of Candida IgG antibodies in patients with medically unexplained symptoms. *J. Altern Complement Med 13:1129-1133*

Using the Fungal Related Disease Questionnaire (FRDQ-7) the researchers selected subjects with a score > 9 and compared Candida IgG antibody concentrations to a control group. The Candida antibody concentrations were significantly higher in the non-control group than in the control group (p<0.001). This is evidence of a real disease and like ABS, it requires more study.

An untold number of patients suffer from organ-related or systemic candida infections and search for relief; but mainstream medicine until recently, largely treated them as concocted illnesses. Finally, the National Institutes of Health now lists Systemic Candidiasis on their rare diseases' website.[108]

••••••

In studying the mycobiome, the same problem arises as with the gut bacteria - The Great Plate Anomaly - meaning nonculturable fungi account for the largest share of the species present in our guts. The two most abundant gut yeast phyla identified thus far are *Ascoymycota* and *Basidomycota*. Humans harbor between five and 39 fungal genera, with an average of fifteen in our oral cavities and from one to nine in our gastrointestinal tract.[109]

I don't mean to belabor the point, but most of what we know about gut microbes, yeast, and fermentation in the gut is a budding science (sorry) and has not made it into mainstream medicine. In order to piece together the constellation of factors in ABS and other yeast-based syndromes, much more research must be done.

Of course, we all see companies that have jumped on the bandwagon to sell, sell, sell, by convincing consumers they must take yet another supplement or processed food product to maintain a healthy gut, or correct constipation. Most of these products have never even been tested on human subjects. We just keep seeing how money drives healthcare advice rather than need and science.

108   National Institutes of Health. Genetic and Rare Diseases Information Center. https://rarediseases.info.nih.gov/diseases/1076/systemic-candidiasis Retrieved 11-9-18

109   Witherden, E. Moyes, D. (2018) Mycobiome and gut inflammation: Implications in gut disease. *Imm Inflam in Health and Disease* https://doi.org/10.1016/B978-0-12-805417-8.00022-6

CHAPTER 8

A GHOST DISEASE: STACEY (PATIENT) AND LARRY (STACEY'S HUSBAND)

If you are not your own doctor, you are a fool.

— *Hippocrates*

I met Larry the same way I met most of the other ABS caregivers I know - through an email. He first contacted me in October of 2016 to ask for information and resources for his wife, Stacey. While dozens of wives, mothers, sisters, and other female caregivers have contacted me, Larry is one of only a few husbands or male caregivers who have reached out.

Stacey's BAC of 542mg/dL or 0.54% is one of the highest ER recorded BACs I have heard of in one of our ABS patients who was still talking and moving. Most doctors consider anything over 0.30% as being potentially lethal and most people at that level would be comatose.

Larry found me through the website and Facebook page, and we talked several times on the phone. I immediately related to him because he had been searching the web and scientific literature for years trying to find a diagnosis for Stacey. He is a scientist at heart and a relentless advocate for his wife.

Larry: *We have spent so much time in and out of ER's - 16 times since 2009. For years, we've been chasing this "ghost" disease you describe in your papers. I always described Stacey's "episodes" as being drunk but not having anything to drink. Everywhere we turned was another dead end or wrong turn with a misdiagnosis.*

Stacey: *I must start by telling you that I was misdiagnosed as a type I diabetic in 2010. I was injecting insulin as prescribed and experiencing many bouts of low-blood sugar. The symptoms of low blood sugar mirror some of those of being intoxicated. I also had been a fairly heavy drinker during this period, so you see, it was hard to put a finger on what symptoms came first.*

After a few months, Larry noticed that I could go days without taking insulin and he insisted on a second opinion. That second doctor said I did not have diabetes.

I can remember one day at home, after I had stopped taking insulin and was not drinking, I kind of "came to" while sitting on the couch. I hadn't fallen asleep, but I felt strange and I could not for the life of me tell you what had happened in the last few hours.

This experience was insane. I would go through patterns of being somewhat "normal" to feeling drunk and not remembering what happened, often injuring myself. Then came the "too drunk", followed by "hangover" accompanied by days of detox symptoms. A few days later, I would finally feel well enough to eat but then the cycle would start over whether I drank or not.

Emotionally this took a huge toll on my life. Everyone assumed I was a fall-down drunk. I stopped socializing altogether. I could not be trusted to take care of my small niece or even my teenage son when my husband was out of town working. I could never commit to plans and had to quit my job altogether. Family vacations were miserable.

I was constantly going to the ER with severe dehydration and seizures. I was arrested in LAX airport for public intoxication when traveling alone to go see my dad in the hospital. I would stay home in my pajamas and had stopped participating in my own life.

Larry: *Stacey's episodes were characterized by stumbling, slurring, delusions and hallucinations and she would have no memory of what had happened. After the misdiagnosis of diabetes, the visits to the ER would only turn up low potassium and she would get infusions and be sent home. The trips to the ER and hospital stays continued and each time she would get her fluids filled back up.*

As far as I know, they never did a BAC, but Stacey told me that one doctor doing an assessment asked how much she drank. When she said, "On occasion", he rolled his eyes. I didn't hear about this incident until years later and I lament the fact I was never told. I feel like if they had given me reason to suspect drinking (such as a high BAC), I may have gone down the ABS path sooner.

In December of 2013, these "episodes" started occurring daily. They always seemed to start late in the day, around 5 or 6PM. If she went to the gym, it would start earlier. She would get to a point of stumbling, falling, getting little to no sleep. During all of this time, she would go to her General Practitioner and they would do blood tests and discover nothing, yet these crashes continued.

Larry on "worst days": There were many "worst" days...the last two years Stacey was sick were qualified to be the worst because every single day, we would argue which was 100% unlike us. I described it to her as "It must be great for you – whatever occurs, you don't remember it and yet every single day, I remember everything." There were days I would throw my clothes into a suitcase to leave and she would talk me out of it... or I would talk myself out of it, knowing if I left, who was going to take care of her?

You would have had to understand the dynamic Stacey and I had before all of this to see how out of character our fighting was. It was draining me to the point I could not take it anymore. I do know if we hadn't caught this when we did, we would either be divorced, separated or she would be dead. Any one of those are a fact.

Stacey: A few years ago, I was asked to be a bridesmaid in a friend's wedding. I had to decline because I had no way of knowing what kind of shape I would be in. I had another friend that had her wedding on the same day. I tried to attend both and barely made it through the ceremony of the first and had to leave before I embarrassed myself and I didn't make it to the second one.

I remember each time I would go through the bouts of throwing up and detoxing that I felt like I was dying. I prayed for death. My diaphragm would be so sore that it hurt to breathe. My throat would be sore from vomiting to the point of not being able to swallow without excruciating pain for days.

Every year we would go to my parents' cabin in Northern Idaho. This was always such a special time for me and my family, but for the last couple of years I was miserable beyond belief: sick, throwing up and missing out on everything. My family was baffled and so worried about me. This will be the first year in a long time that I am able to go.

The quest for a diagnosis was agonizing because often Stacey could not get an appointment with her regular doctor or specialist sooner than six weeks from the time she called. Larry always went to every appointment with her and encouraged the doctors to run more tests and figure out why her potassium was low. He made note of treatments that helped her as well as those that did not. Larry challenged the lack of a diagnosis and insisted on a visit to an Endocrinologist who told them there was nothing wrong with Stacey.

The next stop was to visit a Nephrologist who diagnosed her with Gitelman syndrome. Gitelman syndrome is an inherited salt-wasting (potassium, magnesium and calcium) kidney disease. This doctor tested Stacey and saw low magnesium levels as well as potassium and when they started supplementing both, Larry noticed an improvement in Stacey.

Larry: *But, again, she continued having her crashes. It would get to the point she could not get out of bed or eat because she would vomit for days on end. During the bad ones, she started having grand mal seizures. She had one as recently as March of 2016 and was taken by ambulance to the hospital.*

I started noticing some patterns in her sickness. She also has GERDS and a Hiatal hernia, so heartburn was always a major issue. She was taking Tums or other over-the-counter acid reducers which, as it turns out, sucks magnesium out of you. If she would get stressed, she produced acid and threw up for days. She couldn't keep any food or even her meds down. Sometimes she was able to nurse herself back but there were also many ER visits for potassium and Magnesium.

The other pattern is where she started crashing late in the day, presumably from low electrolytes but her breath was "sweet." For a short period, I was able to test her glucose during one of these crashes. On 3 separate occasions, she measured 152, 175 and 212 blood glucose. To be sure the glucometer was working OK, I tested myself and it came back at 90. So, these crashes happened every day and they began earlier in the day and would get pretty bad. She ended up spending most of her time in bed.

In each case, it was when she went many days of not taking in anything of nutritional value that she had the seizures. There is no tie in with Gitelman Syndrome and seizures that I have found. She had CT scans, MRI's, everything this last time and they found nothing.

Her pattern for several years was get sick, go to ER, get filled up, feel good, start crashing. By this time in 2016, we felt we had nowhere to turn until my wife's United Healthcare nurse suggested we see an Internal Medicine doctor and we started seeing Dr. M.

One of Stacey's issues had been chronic diarrhea which I thought exacerbated her Gitelman Syndrome – remember, we still thought she had this at the time. He immediately took her off prescription Nexium ("It causes diarrhea") and switched to prescription Pepcid. The diarrhea did go away but the frustration that none of the previous 20 doctors we had seen ever caught this was maddening.

Over time with Dr. M., each month they would draw blood and tell her she was low on magnesium. So, we upped the dose of her magnesium supplement and her levels were still low, to the point we were wondering if she was going to need weekly infusions.

Larry on "hope": *The hope for resolution for me came at 2AM the morning of Oct 17, 2016 after an ER visit where she had the .543 BAC. I told the doctors that was impossible as I was with her all night and she had not been drinking. By this time, the staff were basically looking down on us for what they perceived as a closet drinker.*

I had spent the last 9 years trying to do something the doctors could not do – find out what was wrong with my wife. By that time, I could have earned a Medical degree. I recognized the doctors had no vested interest in her since she was just a patient to them, but I had every reason to find the solution to this.

At this point, I am dizzy – dizzy thinking Stacey had been lying to me and the repercussions of that and how I was going to handle this going forward. When she was released, they printed AA information as part of our discharge papers.

On the drive home, we didn't speak as I went back and forth in my head over her possible lying and the hospital being wrong. It was about 1:30 AM when we got home. Once I got her in bed, I searched the house from top to bottom looking for any sign of alcohol. I found nothing – no bottles, no glasses that had remnants or smelled like alcohol – nothing.

Earlier when the ER doctor told me "it's impossible for the body to produce alcohol internally without drinking it. Your wife is a closet alcoholic," I knew in my heart of hearts they were wrong. That is when I did the fateful Google search of "high BAC, no alcohol" and "Gut Fermentation" which led me to Barbara's website and then the Facebook group.

Each and every day, I continued to research what brought me closer to a resolution, which we ultimately found.

Stacey on "worst day" and "hope": *The worst day was when I went to the ER and I had a .543 BAC and the doctors swore up and down that I was a closet alcoholic. But this day was also bittersweet, because it was the day my husband did some research and found information about ABS.*

The day we found your [Barbara's] research on ABS we got a glimmer of hope. Trying to find a doctor that had even heard of it was difficult, let alone one who was willing to treat it. I had gone through so many misdiagnoses and so much hopelessness for so long that just being able to put a label on it was incredibly hopeful.

Thank you for all the work you have done with Auto-Brewery. If it was not for the research you had done, I would still be miserable and hopeless.

Larry on the treatment: *With this information about ABS on hand, we went back to Dr. M. and I told him I believed she is misdiagnosed and does not have Gitelman Syndrome, but instead, Auto Brewery Syndrome. As it turns out gut fermentation studies show low magnesium as part of its symptoms.*

Stacey was in a crashy state and I asked him to do a BAC in addition to blood work. A week later he called and said it was .33 BAC. Our appointment was at 9 AM! He said his practice was not equipped to do the type of work she needed and found us a GI doctor who at least had heard of ABS.

The Facebook group on ABS was instrumental in us not feeling alone during this process and validating that what we had experienced and continued experiencing was what others saw as well.

On our 1ˢᵗ visit to Dr. P., we explained everything and what I had read about, gave him Dr. Cordell's contact info and some places to research ABS. It didn't appear he believed us but was willing to do some studying. He also began testing her BAC with other standard blood work. He had us get a Comprehensive Stool Test to culture for yeast. In addition, he performed an endoscopy to biopsy various places within her digestive tract.

While at that appointment, he said her last blood test showed a .37 BAC – at this point he appeared to get on board with what was going on. He began consulting more with Dr. Kanodia as well as Dr. Cordell. The yeast they found was Candida parapsilosis. She started taking fluconazole (an anti-fungal) in addition to 2 types of probiotics, a candida cleanser with milk thistle, 1000mg of vitamin C and grapefruit seed extract. The milk thistle and vitamin C help the liver process the die off of the candida. After 3 weeks on fluconazole, he switched her to nystatin and monitored her from there.

We went to a no sugar, low carb, no starch diet to help starve the yeast overgrowth. This is not especially easy as many products have hidden sugars in them. But we started having more good days than bad days; only an occasional crash.

Some other anecdotal things we have found are that stress seems to bring on a crash (stress speeds production of alcohol in the body?) and going long periods without eating anything also seems to cause alcohol to generate. I am thinking the body looks for energy and takes from fat which turns it into sugar which then meets yeast and voila, alcohol.

Larry and Stacey have been gracious in sharing their struggle as well as their healing story here. Stacey remains symptom-free after nearly two years and their relationship is mending as well. Larry says their relationship is better than it has ever been. They are also both physically and emotionally healthier now than they were ten years ago.

Larry remains active in the support group discussions and offers a tremendous amount of insight and information to others. Like many of us caregivers, Larry wants to understand more about this disease and help others.

CHAPTER 9 ⌇

GUT DYSBIOSIS AND YEAST OVERGROWTH

Never go to a doctor whose office plants have died.

— *Erma Bombeck*

Now that we understand how complicated our guts are, and what healthy function looks like, let's look at how the processes come together in dysfunction to cause this complicated and savage villain, Auto-Brewery Syndrome. ABS is the intersection of dysfunctional digestion, and over-zealous fermentation by an overgrowth of yeasty beasties. But how does this happen?

Immune dysfunction and disease processes can result when diet, toxins or antibiotics disturb the gut microbiome. Examples include non-alcoholic fatty liver disease (NALFD) and cardiovascular disease.[110] The gut

---

110   Goldsmith J, Sartor R (2014) The role of diet on intestinal microbiota metabolism: downstream impacts on host immune function and health, and therapeutic implications. *J Gastroenterology* 49:785-798. https://doi.org/10.1007/s00535-014-0953-z

microbiome is implicated in inflammatory bowel disease (IBD),[111] irritable bowel syndrome (IBS),[112] metabolic disorders,[113] and obesity.[114]

Even multiple sclerosis, cystic fibrosis, and autism spectrum disorder (ASD) are now linked to a disturbance in the microbiome.[115] ABS is gaining enough discussion and data to be added to the list. Sadly, our diets, medicines, and environment are all contributing to these gut disturbances.

TOO MUCH OF A GOOD THING

The U.S. culture is gripped by a hygienic craze as we disinfect every surface, use sanitizers in place of soap and water, and overuse antibiotics. We've come to think of all bacteria as infectious and we go into a bactericidal frenzy expunging the beneficial microbes as well as the potential pathogens from our food, environment, and bodies.

Repeated antibiotic use is one of the most often described risks for perturbations in the enteric microbiome with resultant *Staph* infections, small intestinal bacterial overgrowth (SIBO), and yes, yeast infections.[116] If you are a woman and got a vaginal yeast infection after taking a course of antibiotics, you now know why.

I was once interviewed about ABS on live radio and while describing yeast in the gut, the DJ asked, "Is that like when my girlfriend gets an

---

111   Kostic A, Xavier R, Gevers D (2014) The microbiome in inflammatory bowel disease: Current status and the future ahead. *Gastroenterology* 146:1489-1499. https://doi.org/10.1053/j.gastro.2014.02.009

112   Jacobs C, Adame E, Attaluri A, Valestin J, Rao S (2013) Dysmotility and proton pump inhibitor use are independent risk factors for small intestinal bacterial and/or fungal overgrowth. *Alimentary Pharmacology and Therapeutics* 37:1103-1111. https://doi.org/10.1111/apt.12304

113   Kovatcheva-Datchary P, Arora,T. (2013) Nutrition, the gut microbiome and the metabolic syndrome. *Best Practice & Research Clin Gastro* 27:59-72. http://dx.doi.org/10.1016/j.bpg.2013.03.017

114   Arora T, Sharma R (2011) Fermentation potential of the gut microbiome: implications for energy homeostasis and weight management. *Nutrition Reviews* 69(2):99-106. https://doi.org/10.1111/j.1753-4887.2010.00365.x

115   Brodin P, Davis M. (2017) Human immune system variation. *Nat Rev Immunol* 17(1):21–29. DOI:10.1038/nri.2016.125

116   Jernberg C, Lofmark S, Edlund C, Jansson J. (2007) Long-term ecological impacts of antibiotic administration on the human intestinal microbiota. *The ISME Journal* 1:56-66. http://www.nature.com/ismej/journal/v1/n1/full/ismej20073a.html

infection in her vajay-jay?" I laughed along with him and said "yes, a vaginal yeast infection is a good analogy."

Most doctors, nurse practitioners, and physician assistants overprescribe antibiotics for the treatment of minor infections, viral infections such as ear infections and flu, and chronic infections such as acne. This habit is now half-a-century old. Of course, we can't lay all the blame on prescribers because many patients and caregivers pressure doctors to give them antibiotics. Some patients feel the doctor didn't do anything for them if he or she didn't prescribe a medication.

The alarming news is that when we repeatedly kill the good bacteria, the setting is ripe for hostile interlopers to attack and over-colonize and even mutate to more lethal pathogens.

The use of anti-bacterial soaps and hand sanitizers in schools, offices, restaurants, and public buildings, coupled with antibiotic use, contribute to the evolution of resistant superbugs such as methicillin-resistant *Staphylococcus aureus* (MRSA),[117] and *Clostridium difficile* (*C. diff*).[118] These superbugs are just what they sound like; mutated super-villains that don't respond to standard antibiotics.

So, if you contract one of these resistant infections, the antibiotics required are extraordinarily potent, hugely expensive, and must be taken in high doses for longer periods of time. The Centers for Disease Control and Prevention (CDC) labels the development of antibiotic-resistant pathogens a crisis that only promises to worsen in the coming years.[119]

The prolific use of antibiotics in the West in cattle and chicken feed contributes to the problem as well. The feed leaves a residual amount of

---

117   Aldeyab M, Scott M, Kearney M, et al. (2014) Impact of an enhanced antibiotic stewardship on reducing methicillin-resistant Staphylococcus aureus in primary and secondary healthcare settings. *Epidemiology and Infection* 142(3):494-50. DOI: https://doi.org/10.1017/S0950268813001374

118   Schubert A, Rogers M, Ring C, et al. (2014) Microbiome data distinguish patients with *clostridium difficile* infection and non-*c. difficile*-associated diarrhea from healthy controls. *MBio* 5(3): DOI:10.1128/mBio.01021-14. https://mbio.asm.org/content/5/3/e01021-14

119   Ventola C. (2015) The antibiotic resistance crisis: Part 1: Causes and threats. *Pharmacy and Therapeutics* 40(4), 277–283

antibiotics in the meat we eat. Federal legislation passed in 2017 outlawed the use of antibiotics in feed on a regular production basis. However, farmers are using a loophole that allows them to use antibiotics for "disease prevention."[120]

Of course farmers want to add antibiotics to feed so their stock gain weight faster or require less food to gain that weight. No one is sure why this works but larger animals certainly draw more money at market; just another example of profit driving an industry instead of health.

••••••

Nearly every ABS patient I've spoken with reports a memorable course of antibiotics just prior to their first ABS attack. Of course, there must be other factors that contribute to ABS or many more people would have it, since most of us received at least one course of antibiotics in our lifetime.

But antibiotics aren't the only disruptors to the microbiome. A recent study in *Nature* from the European Molecular Biology department reported the impact of non-antibiotic drugs on the human microbiome. More than one-fourth (250 out of 923) of the non-antibiotic drugs tested inhibited the growth of at least one strain of gut bacteria found in healthy humans.[121] The drugs included antivirals, antipsychotics, acid-reducing medications, chemotherapy drugs, and blood pressure medications.

Numerous other toxins found in nature can also find their way into our guts and create a disturbance. Bad news for beer drinkers: Dr. Xenia Pascari and her fellow researchers in Spain conducted a survey of mycotoxins in beer. They analyzed 165 beer brands and found that 64 of them contained mycotoxins, with zearalenone being the most abundant.[122] Zearalenone is a major

---

120   Mayer A. (2017) New Federal rules using antibiotics on the farm may fall short. *Harvest Public Media.* http://harvestpublicmedia.org/post/new-federal-rules-using-antibiotics-farm-may-fall-short Retrieved: 11-10-18

121   Maier L, Pruteanu M, Kuhn M, et al. (2018) Extensive impact of non-antibiotic drugs on human gut bacteria. *Nature* 555(7698):623-628

122   Pascari X, Ortiz-Sola J, Marin S, Ramos A, Sanchis V. (2018) Survey of mycotoxins in beer and exposure assessment through the consumption of commercially available beer in Lleida, Spain. *ScienceDirect* 92:87-91. DOI: 10.1016/j.lwt.2018.02021

metabolite of the mycotoxin *a-zearalanol*, a non-steroidal estrogen produced by fungi. So how did Zearalenone find its way into so much of our beer?

The answer is that this compound is abundant in plant material such as hops, that are infected with *Fusarium*. *Fusarium* is a fungus known to cause allergic responses, disseminated infections, and mycotoxicosis in humans and animals.[123] So not only is this toxin disturbing our microbiota, it is linked to allergies, immunosuppression, and infections. Be careful what you drink.

I will tell you that many of our ABS patients reveal a hobby of home brewing or enjoying craft beers and I have often wondered if there is a connection between small amounts of unfermented yeast in the brew and their illness. But maybe, in reality, it's the zearalenone.

••••••

Sulfites are another category of gut disruptor widely used in meats such as sausage and lunch meat, fish, wine, juice, beer, dried fruit and canned goods. Sulfites are toxic additives of sulfur dioxide gas, hydrogen sulfites, metabisulfites, and sulfur salts and can also naturally occur as metabolites in yeast.[124] While sulfites inhibit bacterial contamination in food, they also damage at least four beneficial gut bacteria.[125]

As mentioned in relation to human digestion, typically the sugar by-products of gut fermentation are acids such as propionic acid (PPA) and short-chain fatty acids (SCFA). Generally, medical scientists believe the amount of alcohol fermented in the human intestines to be so low as to be negligible in healthy people. However, a 2014 study by the Max Rubner Institut in Germany

123   Nucci M, Anaissie E. (2007) Fusarium infections in immunocompromised patients. *Clin Micro Rev* Oct.:695-704. DOI:10.1128/CMR.00014-07

124   Leclercq C, Le Donne C, Toledo M. (2009) Sulfites: assessment of dietary exposure. *WHO Food Additive Series* 60:221-244. http://apps.who.int/iris/bitstream/10665/44063/1/9789241660600_eng.pdf Retrieved: 11-9-18

125   Irwin S, Fisher P, Graham E, et al. (2017) Sulfites inhibit the growth of four species of beneficial gut bacteria at concentrations regarded as safe for food. *PLoS. ONE* 12(10): e0186629. https://doi.org/10.1371/journal.pone.0186629

demonstrated that one Lactobacillus species in fecal slurries produced *significant* amounts of ethanol in obese subjects.[126]

Furthermore, it is known that an overgrowth of bacteria produces ethanol at elevated levels in the breath of some patients with end-stage renal disease.[127,128] Ethanol can even be found in otherwise healthy people who have not been drinking. Analytical scientist Dr. Claire Turner and her colleagues in the UK and Czech Republic concluded that "the ethanol levels in the exhaled air are clearly increased after consumption of sugars and action on it by either mouth or gut flora/enzymes."[129]

I recognize the concept of the microbiome is still a mystifying and intimidating force in our health and the threats seem insidious and menacing. Even researchers, doctors, and clinicians can become puzzled by the science, so I know it can be overwhelming to lay people and patients too. Just take it in small parcels the way researchers do – one piece of the puzzle at a time.

Now that we have some insights into what a huge role the gut microbiome plays in the immune system and how easily disturbances to our gut micro- and myco-biomes occur, it makes sense that we are seeing more syndromes, diseases, and auto-immune disorders.

These parallel studies on other diseases add to the scientific plausibility that pathological levels of yeast in the gut mycobiome are indeed causing ABS symptoms. We must bring all the research together to legitimize ABS and bring our scotoma back into medical awareness.

126   Elshaghabee F, Bockelmann W, Meske D, et al. (2014) Modulation of fructose fermentation in fecal slurries obtained from obese subjects by different lactobacilli species. *Max Rubner-Institut*

127   Goerl T, Kischkel S, Sawacki A, et al. (2013) Volatile breath biomarkers for patient monitoring during haemodialysis. *J Breath Research* 7(1). DOI: 10.1088/1752-7155/7/1/017116

128   Rana S, Malik A (2014) Breath tests and irritable bowel syndrome. World Journal of Gastroenterology 20:7587-601. DOI: 10.3748/wjg.v20.i24.7587

129   Turner C, Spanel P, Smith D (2006) A longitudinal study of ethanol and acetaldehyde in the exhaled breath of healthy volunteers using selected-ion flow-tube mass spectrometry. *Rapid Communications in Mass Spectrometry* 20:61-68. https://doi.org/10.1002/rcm.2275

CHAPTER 10 ⌇

LEGITIMIZING ABS

As one patient with chronic fatigue syndrome put it, "The difference between a crazed neurotic and a seriously ill person is simply a test."

— *Maya Dusenbery, Author of Do No Harm*

For the past eight years I've been on a mission to discover the roots of Auto-Brewery Syndrome. Part of the problem is that ABS goes by several other names such as gut fermentation syndrome, abnormal gut fermentation (AGF), alcohol fermentation syndrome, endogenous ethanol fermentation (EEF), drunkenness disease, fungal-type dysbiosis, and gut dysbiosis. And those names are not always found in the titles of published articles.

I am disappointed to find most of the articles on this syndrome are anecdotal case studies rather than controlled research studies. ABS is indeed a medical scotoma; it goes by many names, was identified between the 30s and 70s mostly in non-U.S. publications, and was largely denied, ignored, or forgotten. Only a handful of doctors are now diagnosing ABS, and even fewer are systematically studying the syndrome.

Providers must wake up to the reality of this disorder! They say we are in denial, but they are the ones that refuse to believe ABS exists even when faced with a preponderance of evidence. I once had a doctor ask me why my article wasn't written out of a major university and I responded that the large universities obviously weren't interested. Where *is* the money for research into this rare but debilitating disorder?

As mentioned earlier, Auto-Brewery Syndrome is described as a syndrome whereby patients are intoxicated without ingesting alcohol. All the published cases I've found describe intoxication without drinking as the hallmark symptom. Our 250+ patients corroborate a sudden loss of coordination, slurring words, and passing out without drinking alcohol, or with only a small amount of alcohol. Nearly all of our patients have confirmed their intoxication with a breathalyzer and subsequent blood draws often measuring extremely high alcohol levels.

The published case studies and all the patients diagnosed with ABS I've talked to cite an overgrowth of yeast somewhere in the gut (stomach, small intestine, or large intestine) that ferments carbohydrates into ethanol. Specific yeasts named include: *Candida albicans*, *Candida krusei*, *Candida glabrata*, *Candida kefyr*, and *Saccharomyces cerevisiae*, with *S. cerevisiae* seeming to be the most virulent - as evidenced by our sickest and most intractable patients.[130]

Three of the most recent cases identified four offending pathogens. Dr. Brian Welch and team members from Mayo Clinic found *Candida glabrata* in their case study.[131] Dr. Prasanna Wickremesinghe, affectionately known as Dr. Wick, initially identified *S. cerevisiae*. The patient did not respond to oral antifungals and they later found *Candida Intermedia* as well as the rare growth of *Klebsiella* pneumonia and *Enterococcus faecium* in the Staten Island case.[132] Dr. Xaiodi Guo and his colleagues in Beijing identified *Candida parapsilosis* as the underlying yeast.[133]

130   Cordell B, Kanodia A. (2015) Auto-brewery as an emerging syndrome: Three Representative Case Studies. *J Clin Med Case Reports* 2(2):5. https://doi.org/10.13188/2332-4120.1000013

131   Welch B, Prabhu N, Walkoff L, Trenkner S. (2016) Auto-Brewery Syndrome in the setting of long-standing Crohn's disease: A case report and review of literature. *Journal of Crohn's and Colitis* 10(12):1448-1450. DOI: https://doi.org/10.1093/ecco-jcc/jjw098

132   Ahmed S, Wickremesinghe P, Kopetz V, Sarkar S. (2018) A rare diagnosis of Gut Fermentation Syndrome/Auto-Brewery Syndrome in the setting of diabetes and obesity. *Amer J Clin Path* 150:S2. https://doi.org/10.1093/ajcp/aqy090.003

133   Guo X, Zhang W, Huang R, et al. (2018) The case study of one patient with gut fermentation syndrome: Case report and review of the literature. *Int J Clin Exp Med* 11(4):4324-4329. http://www.ijcem.com/files/ijcem0061289.pdf

THE EARLIEST CASE?

The Welch article claimed the "first case of endogenous alcohol production" was reported in 1948 by Ladkin and Davies with a case of a 5-year-old Ugandan boy. However, Dr. Keith Eaton and Malcolm Howard from England reference an article by J. G. Turner from 1913 expounding "germ carbohydrate fermentation," and a 1931 article by Hurst detailing "intestinal carbohydrate dyspepsia." They go on to say that gut fermentation "enjoyed a popularity in the 1930s and 1940s."[134] Several other authors also referenced the 1913 case as being the earliest.

I located a copy of the 1913 Volume 6 of the Proceedings of the Royal Medical Society and found that Mr. J. G. Turner did not mention intestinal fermentation as referenced. In fact, Robert Saundby, M.D. mentions "auto-intoxication" in another section of the Proceedings where he describes the case of an 18-year-old boy with intoxication due to intestinal fermentation with resulting acetone poisoning.[135] Other authors cite Turner, but this is the risk of citing secondary sources; the primary source states the case is by Saundby.

Saundby ascribes the origin of the doctrine of intestinal auto-intoxication to "Bouchard." The reference must have been well-known at the time because Dr. Saundby does not cite the work. But in fact, Charles Bouchard, a professor of Pathology and Therapeutics in Paris, authored a 368-page tome in 1894 titled *Auto-Intoxication in Disease*, that was translated to English in 1906.[136] In short, it appears science had well-accepted Auto-Brewery in the early 20th Century.

---

134   Eaton K, Howard M. (1998) Fungal-type dysbiosis of the gut: The occurrence of fungal diseases and the response to challenge with yeasty and mould-containing foods. *J Nutr & Envir Med* 8:247-255

135   Saundby R. (1913) A Discussion on Alimentary Toxaemia: its Sources, Consequences and Treatment in: The consequences and treatment of alimentary toxemia from a medical point of view. In Champneys, F.H. Ed. *Proc Roy Soc Med* 6:37-48

136   Bouchard, C. (1906). Lectures on Auto-Intoxication in Disease. Philadelphia: F.A. Davis. https://archive.org/details/lecturesonautoin00bouc/page/n3

MORE SCIENCE

I scoured the literature to find as many post-1950s cases and reports as I could of patients with a documented over-fermenting gut and will summarize them here, but I have also organized a literature review from 1970 to present into a table, *Table of Published ABS Cases,* available on my website: www.autobrewery.info. The table of cases includes the yeast if identified and an underlying pathology if known.

Japanese authors described the best known and most frequently referenced cases of the gut fermentation phenomenon. In 1972, Dr. Kazuo Iwata[137] conducted a review of the literature on what he called 'drunken symptoms' where he states Dr. M. Sato reported the first case in Japan in 1952. So far, I am unable to locate the original Sato article.

Iwata states there were 23 similar cases up to 1972 and he goes on to detail those 24 cases, including the one by Sato, and summarize them in table form. Dr. Iwata credits T. Takasugi and T. Takada in 1960, with coining the phrase *meitei-sho* in Japanese, meaning drunkenness or intoxication (meitei) and disease (sho).

Dr. Iwata recounted the 24 cases where all but one identified an implicated yeast overgrowth. He further found that all but three of the cases identified at least one GI finding such as dilatation, stenosis, reverse peristalsis, or retention of food or contrast medium. He included the treatment of the times for each case in the table as well.

In 1976, Dr. Hiroshi Kaji and his Japanese associates described the case of a 24-year-old female who became intoxicated after consuming carbohydrates which fermented in the gastrointestinal tract.[138] In this woman's situation, cultures determined the causative organisms as *Candida albicans* and *Candida krusei.*

---

137   Iwata K. (1972) A review of the literature on drunken syndromes due to yeasts in the gastrointestinal tract. *Int Spec Symp Yeast,* Tokyo: University of Tokyo Press:260-8

138   Kaji H, Asanuma Y, Ide H, et al. (1976) The Auto-Brewery Syndrome – the repeated attacks of alcoholic intoxication due to the overgrowth of *Candida (albicans)* in the gastrointestinal tract. *Materia Medica Polona* 4(29):429-435

The patient restricted the intake of carbohydrates in her diet and received a course of an antifungal agent. Her intoxication symptoms quickly subsided. This article also used the term *meitei-sho* translated to "Auto-Brewery Syndrome" or "drunkenness disease."

Funny aside: there's a French Afrobeat band named Meï Teï Shô and their music is described as "organic", "takes guts", and "fermented on the roads of France."[139] I'd love to know how they came to choose the name.

Dr. Kaji and other Japanese researchers reported two additional Auto-brewing case studies in an article in 1984.[140] They included a review of 39 cases in table form, including 20 of the cases from Iwata's earlier review. For the additional 19 cases, all but six listed an underlying GI abnormality such as dilatation or stenosis. This was the last article I could find out of Japan.

••••••

In the 2016 case study, Welch mentions the two articles by Hiroshi Kaji and two other cases of ABS with short bowel syndrome and then proceeds to question those cases using a 2000 article by Barry Logan, Ph.D., and Alan Wayne Jones, Ph.D. which summarized older publications on endogenous alcohol.

But wait! Here's the scotoma: Welch, et al. failed to mention the multiple cases cited by the other Japanese authors or the numerous cases of the 1990s published by the Brits with Dr. Keith K. Eaton leading the way. Furthermore, they didn't even acknowledge the handful of case studies published in the 1990s or 2000s.

Dr. Keith Eaton at the Princess Margaret Hospital in Berkshire, England and his colleagues John McLaren Howard, Adrian Hunnisett, and Malcolm Howard, in various combinations, authored at least eight original

139   The World Music Expo. Mei Tei Sho https://www.womex.com/virtual/yotanka_yozik/mei_tei_sho Retrieved 11-12-18

140   Kaji H, Asunuma Y, Yahara O, et al. (1984) Intragastrointestinal Gut Fermentation Syndrome: Report of Two Cases and Review of Literature. *J Foren Sci Soc* 24(5):461-471

articles in the 1990s. They accepted Abnormal Gut Fermentation (AGF) as a legitimate medical issue and conducted research for nearly two decades.

Dr. Eaton and his fellow researchers continued to reprint their articles well into the 2000s. They used the terms "abnormal gut fermentation" and "fungal-type dysbiosis," which probably contributed to the scotoma. John McLaren co-authored an article on yeast dysbiosis as recently as 2005.

One Eaton, et al. study compared 29 subjects with food intolerance to 29 subjects with abnormal gut fermentation (AGF) and to a control group of 50 well individuals. Symptoms overlapped between the AGF and food intolerance, but the two clusters responded differently to an oligo-antigenic diet, also known as an elimination diet.[141]

In another study a clinical test differentiated fermenters from non-fermenters. Of the 53 subjects recruited, 36 were fermenters. The authors were searching for urinary indicators of fermentation but determined that urinary beta-alanine excretion did not vary between the two groups.[142]

Drs. Adrian Hunnisett and John McLaren Howard also of the Princess Margaret Hospital in London, England proposed a clinical test in 1990 to detect dietary fermentation.[143] Subjects suspected of gut fermentation syndrome were given a fasting glucose challenge of 5 Gm glucose orally. One gram of glucose was administered in a hardened gelatin capsule to ensure passage into the duodenum.

Blood glucose levels and blood ethanol levels were then measured at one hour. Fasting blood alcohol levels were zero in nearly all subjects. But 61% of the 510 subjects showed an increase in blood alcohol levels on the average of 2.5 mg/dL (range 1.0 - 7.0 mg/dL). This compared to near zero

---

141   Eaton K, Howard M, Hunnisett A. (1994) Urinary beta-alanine excretion is a marker of abnormal as well as normal gut fermentation. *J Nutr Med* 4(2):157-163

142   Eaton K, Howard M, Howard J. (1995) Gut permeability measured by polyethylene glycol absorption in abnormal gut fermentation as compared with food intolerance. *J Royal Soc Med* 88:63-66

143   Hunnisett A, Howard J. (1990) Gut fermentation (or the 'auto-brewery') syndrome: A new clinical test with initial observations and discussion of clinical and biochemical implications. *J Nutr Med* 1(1):33-39

blood alcohol levels in the control group. Remember this test because there are some problems with it that I'll discuss later in this chapter.

Dr. Janice Joneja, Dr. Elizabeth Ayre, and Kimoko Patterson, of Vancouver Hospital and Health Sciences Centre presented three cases with ABS in a 1997 journal article.[144] They also presented a review of etiology largely predicated on the British researchers Hunnisett and Eaton.

The authors concluded that ABS symptoms present in a similar fashion to food intolerance with the additional symptom of alcohol production. But where ABS patients often respond to antifungal drugs and diet, food intolerance patients do not. They further state that increased permeability of the small intestine is demonstrated in patients with ABS.

I found a handful of reported cases in the last two decades, two of which were identified in children. The first, in 2001 was the case of a 13-year-old girl with short gut syndrome who became intoxicated on multiple occasions.[145] Dr. Ahmed Dahshan and Dr. Kevin Donovan at Oklahoma University Health Science Center published her case.

The doctors suspected her of drinking and so they admitted her to a rehabilitation facility where she would have no access to alcohol. The girl continued to become intoxicated and the doctors connected it to high carbohydrate foods and high fructose juices. They then speculated she might have endogenous fermentation. Aspirates from her small intestines grew *C. glabrata* and *S. cerevisiae*. After treatment with fluconazole, the girl improved.

The other case, in 2006, was a 3-year-old girl in Sweden with short bowel syndrome who became intoxicated after ingesting a fruit drink.[146] Dr. Evelyn Janssen-Nettlebladt and her colleagues at Uppsala University cultured

---

144   Joneja J, Ayre E, Paterson K. (1997) Abnormal gut fermentation: The "Auto-Brewery" Syndrome. *J Canadian Dietetic Assoc* 58(2):97-100

145   Dashan A, Donovan K. (2001) Auto-Brewery Syndrome in a child with short-gut syndrome: Case report and the review of literature. *J Ped Gastroenterology Nutr.* 33:214-215

146   Jansson-Nettelbladt E, Meurling S, Petrini B, Sjo- lin J. (2006) Endogenous ethanol fermentation in a child with short bowel syndrome, *Acta Paediatrica* 95(4):502-504. https://doi.org/10.1111/j.1651-2227.2006.tb02271.x

the gastric fluids and found *C. kefyr* and *S. cerevisiae*. Again, a course of fluconazole eliminated the girl's symptoms.

In 2006, Giulio Spinucci and physician colleagues from Bologna, Italy published yet another case of ABS in a Caucasian man with chronic intestinal pseudo-obstruction.[147] The man was abstinent from alcohol and hospitalized for abdominal pain, belching, and disorientation. *C. albicans* and *S. cerevisiae* were the offending yeast found in his stool and gastric cultures.

The patient had a history of a simple sugar-rich diet and was taking amoxicillin and clavulanic acid (which assists the antibiotic) for SIBO. Twenty-four hours after changing his diet and discontinuing the antibiotic therapy, his blood ethanol returned to zero.

Unlike other cases, the doctors actually reintroduced the amoxicillin, clavulanic acid, and high sugar diet and the patient again produced alcohol. This is an interesting case on two levels: because the man did not require antifungal therapy, and because the authors demonstrated that diet and antibiotics induced the yeast to again ferment.

Physicians, Dr. Andrea Green, Dr. Dean Antonson, and Dr. Kari Simonsen from University of Nebraska Medical Center in Omaha reported a case of ABS in 2012.[148] The patient was a 12-year-old female with a history of short bowel syndrome secondary to omphalocele. She was receiving G-tube feedings and began to experience confusion, dizziness, flank pain, fever, and nausea and vomiting.

On admission, her abdomen was slightly distended, but the rest of the physical examination was unremarkable. The next day when she again experienced confusion and somnolence, her BAC was 208 mg/dL (0.208%). The patient and her parents denied any alcohol consumption. She underwent an EGD and colonoscopy to obtain samples for culture.

---

147   Spinucci G, Guidetti M, Lanzoni E, Pironi L. (2006) Endogenous ethanol production in a patient with chronic intestinal pseudo-obstruction and small intestinal bacterial overgrowth. *Euro J Gastro & Hep* 18:799-802. DOI: 10.1097/01.meg.0000223906.55245.61

148   Green A, Antonson D, Simonsen K. (2012) Twelve-year-old female with short bowel syndrome presents with dizziness and confusion. *Pediatr Infect Dis J* 31:425-430

The bacterial growth of *Enterococcus faecium* from her small bowel and *Enterobacter cloacae,* and *E. faecium* from her colon was consistent with SIBO. The yeast growth of *C. glabrata* from her small bowel and *C. glabrata* from her colon along with her alcohol level confirmed a diagnosis of Auto-Brewery Syndrome.

The patient took a course of fluconazole and then voriconazole, followed a lower carbohydrate diet, and had no further symptoms of ABS. However, six months later she had another abdominal surgery and three months after that, she relapsed with alcohol levels of 390 mg/dL. This time, the offending yeasts were *Citrobacter freundii* and *Candida glabrata.* The article does not detail her treatment for the relapse.

Then there are the two case study articles I co-authored on Auto-Brewery Syndrome. The first article was written with Dr. Justin McCarthy, who diagnosed and treated my husband, Joe, after reading the research we gave him.[149] I called Joe "a friend" in the article because at that point he wanted to be anonymous. While the medical course is detailed here, you heard the visceral story (groan) from Joe and me in Chapter 3.

Dr. McCarthy followed the protocol for a 24-hour hospital observation to diagnose ABS. Once he was convinced of the diagnosis, the doctor prescribed a course of anti-fungal medication, along with a low carbohydrate diet and probiotics. Thankfully, Joe responded and has been symptom-free for nearly nine years.

Dr. Anup Kanodia worked with me on the second article[150] after he diagnosed ABS in a dozen or so patients who contacted us. Together, we selected three cases representative of the spectrum of cases he was treating with varying levels of success. The first case was a 60-year-old man with a four-year history of drunkenness without drinking. He was a recovering alcoholic with 23 years of abstinence from alcohol.

---

149   Cordell B, McCarthy, J. (2013). A case study of gut fermentation syndrome (auto-brewery) with *Saccharomyces cerevisiae* as the causative organism. *International Journal of Clinical Medicine* 4:7. Article ID:33912, 4 p. Open Access: http://file.scirp.org/Html/1-2100535_33912.htm

150   Cordell B, Kanodia A. Ibid.

This patient's drunken symptoms began after a fall and hospitalization. He sought information from me and treatment from Dr. Kanodia in the autumn of 2014. His stool cultures showed *C. albicans* and *C. krusei*, and the patient was given a course of nystatin. He was prescribed a strict diet and was counseled to avoid mold and seemed to be responding to treatment.

However, when he returned to his trucking job hauling grain, his symptoms returned. Dr. Kanodia believes the mold in the grain stirred up the ABS again and he recommended the patient change jobs, if possible. By summer of 2015 this man had lost 40 pounds, no longer had symptoms of intoxication and was working again, but not hauling grain. This case shows how difficult it can be to identify and eliminate triggers.

The second case was a 42-year-old woman from Georgia with a several-year history of drunken episodes. She had been to internists, psychologists, psychiatrists, and neurologists without finding a diagnosis. Her partner contacted me, and I referred her to Dr. Kanodia. I stayed in touch with them to help answer questions and collect additional information.

This patient and her partner kept an excellent diary of food, activity, and episodes. One entry stated: *Days that involve a lot of stress, running around, and mental energy almost always end with an episode. Mondays through Wednesdays are her busiest days and were almost guaranteed to result in episodes. On the weekends, when she was relaxed and less stressed, she was less likely to become intoxicated.*

The patient's stool tested positive for *S. cerevisiae* and *S. bulardii* and she was given a course of the antifungal fluconazole but still had positive stool cultures. She was put on a low carbohydrate diet, but had difficulty complying and was referred to a nutritionist. The patient was counseled on a very strict diet, along with supplements and probiotics. She improved dramatically and reported feeling much better.

This case represents the difficulty in finding the right combination of treatments for an individual patient. She required a combination of conventional and integrative treatments to find relief. The patient reported being symptom-free for two years but then we lost track of her.

The third and final case in our article was the difficult case of Nick, who you read about in Chapter 6. Nick represents the challenge of treating ABS when it becomes chronic. He continues to relapse with ABS and may have other underlying diseases. His search continues.

......

The previously mentioned 2016 Welch article[151] describes the case of a 71-year-old man with Crohn disease. The patient had a history of a small bowel resection decades prior with a recent history of repeated courses of antibiotics for diarrhea. The doctors found the presence of *C. glabrata* in the stool and stopped antibiotics, treating the patient with diet instead.

The mechanism of ABS proposed by Dr. Brian Welch and his colleagues is that the distended bowel "acted like a 'vat' and...increased sugar intake acted as the substrate for fermentation (p.2)". This has significant implications for all patients with symptoms of ABS. Maybe there is some distension in other ABS patients that creates that vat!

Dr. Xaiodi Guo and Dr. Weiyan Zhang, department of infectious disease, and other physicians in Beijing published an ABS case study in early 2018.[152] They describe the diagnosis of ABS as "time consuming and dramatic". Their case is a 30-year-old male who suffered for years from severe episodes of intoxication and vomiting without drinking. He had elevated liver enzymes and regularly received IV hepatoprotective infusions.

The patient was also diagnosed with nervous vomiting and prescribed Sertraline and Alprazolam for six months without improvement. When he presented in 2013, he was strictly monitored and ultimately diagnosed with gut fermentation syndrome with a BAC of 311.2 mg/dL or 0.31%. His two stool samples identified an overgrowth of *C. parapsilosis*.

The patient took fluconazole and "Bifico six tablets per day" (a probiotic) and improved significantly. However, he still had mild episodes intermittently, so he then took voriconazole and nystatin along with a low

---

151   Welch B, et al. Ibid.

152   Guo X, et al. Ibid

carbohydrate diet. The patient experienced relief once he completed the regimen and remained symptom-free from 2016 until the article was published.

Dr. Anup Kanodia, Dr. Greg Miller, and I completed a case-controlled research study in 2018 accepted for publication in 2019 by Global Advances in Health and Medicine.[153] We administered a 78-item questionnaire to 28 ABS patients and 18 family members to try and determine common medical history, health, lifestyle, and diet factors that should be examined more closely.

The showed the patients with ABS have statistically significant differences compared to people without ABS in lower quality bowel movements, more frequent bowel movements, more reports of malodorous breath, and self-classify as having poorer health. Furthermore, the ABS folks consume more water, less tea and coffee, fewer dairy products, less candy, eat out less and rely on food prepared at home. They also have more aversion to starch, and more food sensitivities than the group without ABS.

The ABS group reports more diarrhea, higher amounts of yeast in their GI tract, and using acne medication for a longer time than the control group. We concluded that patients with ABS have significant differences in their lifestyle and health, diet, and past medical history compared to non-ABS participants and these differences warrant further research.

We have a second set of data comparing the combined research group on the survey to the set of data from the American Gut Project. We hope to publish these data soon to add to the knowledge we have about ABS.

You'll read about the Staten Island case in the next chapter. Donato suffered multiple symptoms of intoxication and other maladies. His doctors have since treated at least seven other patients with ABS and published Donato's case in 2018 in the American Journal of Clinical Pathology.[154] Drs. Ahmed, Wickremesinghe, and two other physicians described his diagnosis

---

153   Cordell, B., Kanodia, A., and Miller, G. (2019). Case control research study of Auto-Brewery Syndrome. *Global Advances in Health and Medicine.* 8:1-7. https://doi.org/10.1177/2164956119837566

154   Ahmed S, et al. Ibid.

with ABS and the difficulty tracking down the contributing pathogens and Donato's ultimate treatment with IV antifungal medication.

As mentioned, I have summarized the modern cases on Auto-Brewery Syndrome and its other appellations on my website: www.autobrewery.info. The list is a work in progress, so if you know of any other published cases of ABS I've missed, please let me know at: autobrewery@gmail.com

•••••••

Okay, parents, listen to this one: bacteriologists combined five infant food formulas and supplements with four common gut yeasts (*C. albicans*, *C. tropicalis*, *Torulopsis glabrata*, and *S. cerevisiae*) to measure alcohol production.[155] They incubated the mixtures at 98.6 degrees F. in the lab to mimic body temperature.

All the mixtures of yeast and carbohydrate produced ethanol with the *S. cerevisiae* preparations being the highest. The authors suggest this could be an explanation for ABS. Just think of the implications of this information as formula reaches your baby's gut! Yet another reason to breast feed.

I found three other articles that do not name a specific syndrome but discuss abnormal or unusual fermentation. One was in relation to high fiber diets,[156] another the use of ampicillin,[157] and the third the ingestion of prebiotic inulin.[158]

Even with all the cases and information in the literature, a huge mystery still surrounds the rare syndrome know as auto-brewery. What we know is that in some people a yeast that normally exists quite happily in the gut

155   Bivin W, Heinen G. (1985) Production of ethanol from infant food formulas by common yeasts. *J Appl Bacter* 58(4):355-357. DOI:10.1111/j.1365-2672.1985.tb01473.x

156   Fleming S, Marthinsen D, Kuhnlein H. (1983) Colonic function and fermentation in men consuming high fiber diets. *J Nutr* 113(12):2535-2544. http://jn.nutrition.org/content/113/12/2535.full.pdf+html?sid=ca1b1840-1887-4cc6-936d-1844793aa52c

157   Rao S, Edwards C, Austen S, Bruce C, Read N. (1988) Impaired colonic fermentation of carbohydrate after ampicillin. *Gastro* 94(4):928-932

158   Sauer J, Richter K, Pool-Zobel B. (2007) Products formed during fermentation of the prebiotic inulin with human gut flora enhance expression of biotransformation genes in human primary colon cells. *Brit J Nutr* 97(5):928-938. DOI:10.1017/S0007114507666422

grows out of control over time and ferments the starches and sugars from food into alcohol.

When enough alcohol is produced by the yeast, the poor patient becomes intoxicated. We also know that patients with ABS have a disturbed gut microbiome possibly from antibiotics or toxins that allowed the abundant overgrowth of yeast in the gut.

What we do not know is why one person develops ABS and another does not. We also don't know why some patients respond readily to known treatments and others do not. Families who have a loved one that continues to struggle with symptoms would be overjoyed to find the underlying connections because the knowledge might lead to better treatments.

Might people with ABS also have abnormalities in enzyme production that control fermenting yeast? Birth defects such as congenitally shortened bowels? Or genetic or functionally slowed transit time? Or a combination of factors?

Gastroparesis, or slowed intestinal motility, is a well-known condition with unknown causes and can produce nausea, vomiting, and cause problems with blood sugar levels and nutrition.[159] Could this condition in combination with other issues lead to ABS?

ARGUMENTS AGAINST ABS

Some physicians and attorneys argue against the existence of ABS as a syndrome because they realize that a known quantity of glucose in the presence of fermenting yeast produces a known quantity of ethanol in a controlled environment.

In an article published in 2000, J. A. Gatt and P. Matthewman, dispute the test described by Hunnisett and Howard that administers 5gm of glucose to the patient.[160] They argue that the variable ranges and higher levels of

---

159   Mayo Clinic. Gastroparesis. https://www.mayoclinic.org/diseases-conditions/gastroparesis/symptoms-causes/syc-20355787 Retrieved 8-20-18

160   Gatt J, Matthewman P. (2000) Autobrewing: fact or fantasy? *Sci & Justice* 40(3):211-215

elevated blood alcohol such as .12% or even .04% as reported in case studies are evidence that a person cannot be fermenting. They state, it is "theoretically impossible to attain a blood alcohol level of 19 mg% from the ingestion and fermentation of 5 g glucose."

But, guess what? The human body is non-theoretical! Gatt and Matthewman do not take into account the delayed fermentation of food previously ingested that is further along the intestinal tract where most fermentation occurs. And neither did Hunnisett, for that matter. Many of our patients report their symptoms appearing hours or even a day or two after a high-carbohydrate meal.

For some of our patients, a small amount of potatoes, ice cream, or soda seems to 'kick start' the fermentation of foods already in the pipeline. Many patients were tested for yeast in various locations throughout the intestinal tract. Their doctors found yeast in the small intestines for some and in the large intestines for others. It seems the Hunnisett test is inaccurate because it relies only on fermentation from the duodenum, which is the beginning of the small intestine and takes a measurement within an hour.

Here's more evidence of the scotoma: authors Gatt and Matthewman, of *Autobrewing: fact or fantasy?* are from the United Kingdom. They strangely ignored the other numerous articles published out of England besides Hunnisett and really all the medical cases. They chose instead to focus only on four cases where Auto-Brewery was used as a defense for driving while intoxicated.

Two of the cases were women who decided to drop their defenses. The other two cases were men who agreed to submit to testing under controlled conditions. Both produced endogenous alcohol and their defense attorneys made the case for ABS as the cause. In both cases, the procedures and scientific validity of the testing were questioned as well as the "expected" ratio of glucose to ethanol and the subjects were found guilty.

They then referenced the article by Hunnisett et al. about the testing protocol, and then refuted that protocol. Based on these four cases, Gatt and

Matthewman concluded there is not "any additional evidence that the phenomenon of autobrewing can exist in healthy individuals..." (p. 215). Wait; whoever said people with ABS are healthy? And how can two cases warrant a conclusion when they themselves question the method of testing?

They didn't even look at the evidence. Sadly, many prosecutors still rely on this older article in seeking DUI convictions and dismissing the medical fact of auto-brewing.

I was unable to find any other articles published by either Gatt or Matthewman before or since 2000. Furthermore, I could not locate their profiles at their institutions or on professional author websites. Okay Gatt and Matthewman, come out of hiding and back up your claims, or the rest of the world should ignore your old article.

••••••

Forensic scientists also argue against the plausibility of ABS due to the amount of carbon dioxide (CO_2) produced by the commercial process of fermentation. They want to know where all the CO_2 produced in humans goes. Yes, during a controlled process of fermentation a measurable amount of CO_2 is produced - one molecule of ethanol to one molecule of CO_2.

The volume of gas depends on temperature and pressure. In the brewing industry, calculations of ethanol are made based on the amount of CO_2 produced at *Standard Temperature and Pressure (STP)* of 0° Celsius or 32° Fahrenheit (F.) and 1 atmosphere. The chemists in these situations also know the volume of the starting culture.

What the forensic folks fail to acknowledge is that the human body is not anything like the controlled brewing process used for wine, beer, or other spirits. First, the temperature is not 32° F. but hovers around 98.6° F. In humans, pressure can increase as a result of flatus, including the production of CO_2, nitrogen, methane and other gases, causing discomfort and pain. We know that about 30% of the CO_2 produced normally is reabsorbed by the body.

Our ABS sufferers report enormous amounts of gas and resultant eructation (isn't that a great word for belching?) and flatus (farts). Perhaps they also absorb more than the average 30%? I can't fathom the design of a research study to test gas in a human body with ABS, but we nonetheless must stop using only bench science to explain human physiology.

••••••

The United Arab Emirates would be a terrible place to develop ABS. The country has zero tolerance of alcohol with no allowed legal limit. I mentioned this study earlier, but let's look at it again because it's being used to refute the existence of ABS.

Because four scientists at the Forensic Science Laboratory in Abu Dhabi, UAE realized that small amounts of fermentation of alcohol may occur in all of us, they studied 1557 average residents in 2004 to determine fermentation rates.[161] The subjects represented 13 nationalities and both males (944) and females (613).

The authors conclude that fermentation of ethanol was "too low to have any forensic significance" (p. 149). However, it is important to note that the when the data were pooled (combined without being weighted), the maximum blood alcohol level was 3.52 mg/dL (0.0035%) in males and 3.20 mg/dL (0.0032%) in females, not zero.

These forensic scientists failed to seek out the rare people who have been diagnosed with fermentation dysbiosis; they only selected "average people." I find their conclusion frightening because they use it to "confirm" that ABS is not real.

••••••

Dr. Barry Logan and Dr. Alan Wayne Jones, toxicologists from Washington and Sweden respectively, judge the accounts of Japanese ABS cases as

---

161   Al-Awahdi A, Wasfi I, Reyami F, Al-Hatali Z. (2004) Autobrewing revisted: Endogenous concentrations of blood ethanol in residents of the United Arab Emirates. *Sci & Justice*. 44:149-152

"reliable" and state, "this syndrome...has only ever been documented in Japanese people."[162] What? More scotoma!

This article was published in 2000 and completely ignored the numerous articles published out of England by Eaton, Howard, and Hunnisett, as well as other physicians documenting dozens of cases of gut fermentation throughout the 1980s and 1990s.

Many of the arguments against Auto-Brewery Syndrome assume that the patients in these cases are "otherwise healthy," as Gatt and Matthewman suggest. We aren't claiming that our patients are healthy. And most of them are not trying to fight a legal battle; they just want to be diagnosed and treated so they can be well. Are these lawyers or lab technicians trying to debunk ABS for an ulterior motive? Perhaps they just want to enforce punishment for drunk drivers without dealing with doubt.

We know that ABS patients have yeast overgrowth, but they may also have one or more underlying health challenges including leaky gut (increased intestinal permeability), gastroesophageal reflux disease (GERD), shortened bowel, delayed transit time (gastroparesis), enzyme deficiencies, ALDH issues, SIBO, and possibly a combination of those or other conditions.

Most of our patients just want to get better so once the medication and diet works, we seldom talk to them again. We encourage more providers to publish ABS case studies that examine comorbidities that could shed light on ABS diagnosis and treatment. Also, the forensic and medical arguments need to be brought up to date with current science, thereby acknowledging our scotoma so people can be treated appropriately and with compassion.

---

162   Logan B, Jones A. (2000) Endogenous ethanol "Auto-Brewery Syndrome" as a drunk-driving defence challenge. *Medical Science Law* 40(3):206-216

CHAPTER 11

FOR BETTER OR WORSE: DONATO (PATIENT) AND MICHELLE (DONATO'S WIFE)

"It is far more important to know what person the disease has than what disease the person has."

— *Hippocrates*

Michelle first contacted me in November of 2016, and she was a ball of fire! I certainly met my match for searching literature and I have learned at least as much from Michelle as she has learned from me.

Her then 44-year-old husband-to-be, Donato, had surgery in September 2015. He developed a post-op infection and received IV and oral antibiotics. Since that time, he had been suffering from diarrhea, swelling, seizures, vomiting, blackouts, hallucinations, and intermittent fever and chills. He experienced uncontrolled blood pressure and blood sugar, slept a lot, gained significant weight, and was on oxygen. He had no diagnosis other than complications from Type II diabetes.

Michelle had been searching for clues when she found our article about Joe, emailed me and asked if I could call her. We talked on the phone for hours over the subsequent months because Michelle believed Donato had ABS. We shared our horror stories and forged a friendship built on our common mission to find answers about this crazy syndrome.

In the ABS support group, Michelle asked every question she could think of to help her make sense of what they were going through. She and

Donato went to their Gastroenterologist with case studies and a journal of his BAC readings and the doctor followed the Cordell-McCarthy protocol. Within 45 minutes of admitting Donato for a 24-hour observation, his BAC went from zero to 0.238% and he was diagnosed with ABS.

Even though Donato's stool tests were then negative, the doctor followed the case study protocol by giving him medication. But Donato was still flaring. He needed more than the previous protocols could offer.

Michelle expanded her search for a doctor using www.grandrounds. com and only found one doctor in Boston who had heard of ABS but had never treated anyone. She could not comprehend that there wasn't a doctor in the Tri-State Area to treat Donato. I sent her every reference article I had, and she took them to doctor after doctor. Talk about a call to action; she wasn't taking "no" for an answer.

Donato: Early days: *It's a horrible feeling to be fine one minute and wake up the next to find you have tubes in you. How weird it is to wake up restrained, and to be accused of drinking alcohol.*

I don't remember much about the first seizure in November 2015. It was Halloween and we were giving out candy to the kids trick or treating. We had friends over, had dinner together, and we were eating some of the Halloween candy. The next morning, my wife found me in bed having a seizure while on my back, and I was vomiting. I was choking on my own vomit. She had enough strength to turn me over, so I would not suffocate. BOOM, the next day I woke up in the hospital.

I had no idea; I learned later that I passed out, woke up in the hospital and had tubes in me and I was restrained. That got me more pissed because, yeah, these tubes are gonna keep me alive but, still, it was very irritating, and I tried to pull them out. And, honestly, to this day, I just don't feel right; I feel there's something rasping in my throat. It's been two years now and it still doesn't feel right.

I was in the ICU for a week, and doctors kept asking if I drank alcohol. I didn't. Doctors could not understand why my body was in alcohol withdrawal - neither could we. Michelle called my family to let them know I was in the hospital. My family thought I was going to die. So, they all came to say "goodbye." It was horrible.

Michelle kept a logbook of my symptoms prior to diagnosis and started a binder and kept all the paperwork – EKG, bloodwork, and just continued. Y'know, any new doctor you see, they always want to start over at 'A,' but she kept the paperwork, so they could see what had already been done.

The second [seizure] was Christmas Eve, 2015. We were having dinner at my mother's house. It was sometime after midnight that my mother found me on the bathroom floor having a seizure and she called 911.

Michelle: Thanksgiving 2016: *The stars were aligned Thanksgiving weekend 2016. I decided to visit with my Aunt in Long Island, NY, and my mother was there visiting from Florida. My doctor cousin and his wife, also a doctor, decided to drop by and we all had dinner together. My cousins were concerned about my husband's rapidly declining health. They wanted to know what was going on.*

I described everything we had been through for the past year, including doctors telling me that his body was in alcohol withdrawal. My cousin's wife had just attended a medical conference for rare and unusual conditions and Auto-Brewery Syndrome was one of the topics. We googled it and found the publication by Barbara Cordell. We realized my husband fit the profile.

The next day we purchased an alcohol meter online and I had it shipped overnight. At the same time, I called his Pulmonologist and asked for a GI doctor to see right away. The Pulmonologist told the GI doctor my husband was very sick and needed to be seen immediately. We had an appointment two days later.

I researched the information on the Internet and printed everything I could on ABS. I talked to Barbara and joined the support group to learn all I could. The doctors had never heard of ABS but the GI believed us because of the overwhelming medical information we collected and logged for the last 14 months. He admitted my husband to the hospital on 12/9/16, and with high carb foods, we were able to prove in a supervised medical setting that my husband had ABS.

Having a confirmed diagnosis gave us so much hope. We called every single one of our doctors and told them that we were able to reproduce the alcohol with food in a hospital setting. None of our doctors had heard of this - they all believed it - but none knew what to do. I figured we lived so close to NYC - how hard could it possibly be to cure this? Boy, were we ever wrong!

Donato: [Once the ABS was diagnosed], *it was such a relief. You have no idea. Because before that, I would go to work (I don't sleep much), and get to work an hour or two early, relax in my car in the parking lot, drink coffee, and one day they don't see me at work. Nobody ever said, "go look in his car," and I was passed out in the car. God forbid I was involved in an accident, I mean, how could you explain that? Or God forbid, hurt somebody, have that on your conscience?*

When I finally got diagnosed it was a relief, then it was more frustrating to run into closed doors, meaning doctors. How many doctors did we call and make appointments with and were told no?

I was hospitalized 22 times - the IV's, the x-rays, the oxygen tanks, the blood tests, the scans, the EKGs - constantly someone poking me with some kind of needle for a test. My arms were black and blue and sore. They didn't heal before I was back in the hospital and they were looking for a new vein.

Most of the time, like 90%, I didn't think I was going to survive this. I thought I was going to die. I had tubes down my throat, I had central lines to my heart, I was always connected to some kind of tube, medicine and oxygen. I did not think I was going to live.

Michelle: March 2017 in various support group posts: *This morning he woke up with a blood sugar of 307 and BAC of 0.14. I'm going out of my mind. We have 0 to .33 in 2 hours twice a day. WHAT is going on? No food or beverage consumed. His sugar never drops. It's always around 140 or above. He does eat protein, no carbs when he is awake - the problem I'm having these days is him staying awake.*

I'm under such severe stress that I am having tightness in my chest and shortness of breath. I went to my Dr. and he did an EKG - confirmed it is just stress. Donato has not been able to go to work for days. We just got a prescription for fluconazole for 3-weeks - hopefully that will make a dent. He did good back in De.c and Jan. on the Diflucan (fluconazole). He was able to go to work and his BAC was manageable in the PM.

Getting off the probiotics for one week in preparation for a breath overgrowth test spiraled him backwards, so we are starting over. At least we know more now than we did in December, so hopefully this day going forward we will be able to finally reverse this.

Two questions for anyone that was on the fluconazole and nystatin: How long did it take to get reasonable readings with alcohol levels while on fluconazole? My boyfriend completed four full days and just took the fifth dose. His BAC was zero this morning and stayed that way until four hours after he ate breakfast, then it shot up to .33. Then it started dropping to .17 in about an hour or so and then two hours later shot back up to .33.

My boyfriend's blood glucose and BAC continues to shoot up to 450+ and .33[%] every night between 4pm - 6pm. Every single night. Doesn't matter - with food, without, and he's not eating carbs at all. Is it possible that whatever yeast/fungus he has may have reached his blood stream?

They gave him enough medication and his BAC numbers were starting to drop but he was still flaring. The doctor said we should seriously consider cancelling the wedding. I said, 'We have time to cancel the wedding, let's get through this ordeal.'

Just before April 16th which was Easter Sunday, they wanted to do a colonoscopy and endoscopy. I asked if they could wait until after Easter dinner and they said 'yes'. After the procedure the doctor said, "I hand-carried the samples directly to the head of the lab!" We were so nervous but knew the results could take a while to come back.

An online news outlet picked up on Michelle and Donato's story. Here is an excerpt from the article, *For Better or For Worse* --Kristin Dalton, Staten Island Live; https://www.silive.com/news/2017/08/drunk_without_drinking_a_drop.html

As the illness continued to progress, there was a major event to deal with: Donato [Danny] and Michelle were in the middle of planning their wedding. "Two weeks prior, I met with our vendors and told them I can't guarantee he's going to be here for this wedding and I'm freaking out," Michelle recalled. She said all of the vendors were more than understanding and told her if she had to cancel last minute -- even up until the night before the wedding -- they wouldn't charge her a cent. "It was such a relief -- we didn't buy wedding insurance," she said.

Donato barely made it through the wedding. He was vomiting for hours before and after the ceremony and blacked out as soon as they made it back to their hotel room. But Michelle was at his side throughout it all --- for better and for worse. They tied the knot on April 29, 2017. But the quest for a cure continued.

Michelle: 5-1-17: *Right after the wedding on April 29, 2017, he was admitted for pancreatitis and we had to cancel our honeymoon. At this point the doctors were talking about fecal transplants and admitted him to ICU.*

5-10-17 post to support group: *He is out of ICU and moved into a regular room. After three courses for 21 days each of Diflucan, the first two courses at 100mg and the third at 200mg, no improvement.*

Remember the colonoscopy and endoscopy with cultures back in April? The Colonoscopy proved he has Saccharomyces cerevisiae. We've been waiting for the cultures from the endoscopy, and the lab called and said, "things are starting to bud." It came back Candida Intermedia which was resistant to Diflucan!!

The infectious disease doctor felt there may also be more yeast growing in him that the cultures did not show, so she started him on micafungin sodium via I.V. Since then, he lost 22 lbs. of swelling alone, his blood sugar returned to normal and his blood alcohol is zero from .39. I will have him re-test after dinner tonight to make sure it's still zero.

Between the GI Doctor and the Infectious Disease doctor, they are working together to identify the source and kill it. I cannot believe how quickly he improved - it's dramatic. Almost overnight improvement.

This is the best response to medication so far but we're both walking on eggshells thinking, "What if this doesn't work?" We're cautiously optimistic and feel we finally have the right team of doctors that communicate with us and each other; they are determined to reverse Donato's ABS.

It's sometimes hard for Donato to assess how he feels because when he flares, he has memory blackouts. This week he asked if he was okay; did anything happen the night before? When I told him he was okay, he was so relieved. We have hope that this medication finally will be the one that works.

Today they installed a PICC [peripherally inserted central catheter] line in preparation for sending him home. He will be on a four-week antibiotic course with the PICC line. The infectious disease [doctor] said she feels the reason why the Diflucan didn't work is because he has something else brewing that we did not yet identify.

All the doctors at the hospital are looking at Barbara Cordell's publications and reaching out to her. Since I started this journey, I learned of two more people that have this where I live. I told the doctors and they were shocked to learn about the other two cases. I told them, this is not rare, it's rarely diagnosed.

Donato to Michelle: *When you have ABS, you feel frustrated, helpless, and angry. I don't like it when I have to be taken care of - I'm supposed to be the one that takes care of you, and provides, not the other way around.*

When you first videoed me to show me what I was like, before we even knew what this was, and played it for me when I was…oh, I was shocked. I really understood why you were so concerned. But I was also embarrassed that you filmed me. I did not like seeing myself like that, that's why I asked you never to video me again.

You would ask me the next morning if I had remembered anything from the night before, and it was painful to watch you cry when I told you I didn't. I knew you were telling the truth, but I did not want you to be upset.

I have no control over this. I never felt the flares coming on. One minute I am fine, and then the next I'm not, and when I was not, I had no idea. I didn't know until you told me the next morning.

I hate not being in control of this. It's very draining, and you are very tired. I think if I was someone who drank regularly it would have been better, because I could have made a conscious decision to stop drinking or not drink. This is different.

Michelle: 5-20-17: *My husband's cultures yielded yeast throughout his intestines and stomach. They restored him back to "normal" and gave him meds for alcohol withdrawal when he was on the anti-fungal micafungin sodium via IV.*

Yesterday they took his PICC line out and put a new one in his arm, and today he was sent home. We have a visiting nurse coming tomorrow morning to show us how to do the medicine ourselves. According to the infectious disease doctor, the micafungin is an all-inclusive yeast and fungus killer. Diflucan may not kill everything and that's why it didn't work for him.

Michelle: 6-10-17: *He has completed his 4th week of the yeast IV medication (micafungin Sodium) and most of the time his BAC is 0. The endoscopy revealed that he has two different bacteria in his stomach that don't belong there: Klebsiella and Enterococcus Faecalis. The doctors don't want to treat the bacteria yet - they don't want to complicate things. We also were told that the correct yeast that was identified in his body was Candida Intermedia.*

Donato may have to stay on the IV micafungin another 4-6 weeks then possibly start on two antibiotics to kill the bacteria in his stomach. The doctors are following this case closely ordering weekly blood tests; we are all just playing mad scientist until we see "normal."

Michelle: 6-14-17: *My husband still has the PICC line in his arm to his chest. He still administers the micafungin sodium IV drip every night. We are on week seven. This was the fix for us. He no longer produces alcohol. He eats everything; animal and plant protein, rice, bread, pasta, potatoes, all green veggies, dairy -* NO REACTION.

We are so relieved. At first, we were alarmed that the published protocols did not work for Donato; but our doctors picked a medication that is not in any other case study and it's working for him. The doctors think that when taking samples during a colonoscopy and endoscopy, they might have missed other brewing yeast which is why the previous medicines didn't work.

This was the cure for us. He was too overloaded with yeast for holistic remedies to work. He needed the IV for weeks before it started working, and now it looks like he's completely reversed. His blood sugars have also normalized.

The doctors are not in a rush to take out the PICC line and stop the micafungin IV drip until the results of the endoscopy are back, and they do another colonoscopy culture. We will find out hopefully this Tuesday when his colonoscopy will be scheduled. Once the culture results show "all clear," the PICC line will be removed.

Michelle: 6-27-17: *My husband's endoscopy results: no yeast, no bacteria. One more week of the micafungin sodium and then the PICC line comes out around 7/5/17. Colonoscopy will be scheduled for next week and we expect no more yeast. It's such a relief to be able to cook a normal meal for Donato.*

Donato: *I really missed regular food. From December 2016 to July 2017 I had NO carbs. I was frustrated when we went to restaurants; I'd watch as the waiters would bring "regular" food to other customers. I longed to eat normal and now I can. I am getting my life back. My blood sugars and swelling is better and I can go back to work. I hated that Michelle had to do most everything while I was sick.*

Donato has been symptom free since this last episode. His liver and kidney counts have returned to normal, as well as his potassium, magnesium, and pancreatic levels. He tries to stick to a low to moderate carbohydrate diet, no alcohol and his blood sugar is starting to normalize. He takes a daily probiotic with at least 11 different strains, primarily lactobacillus, with a *minimum* CFU count of 100 billion.

Donato has regular checkups with his team of medical professionals; Dr. Wick, Gastroenterologist, Infectious Disease, Endocrinologist, Pulmonologist, and Nephrologist as well as his licensed nutritionist. He is monitored closely with blood tests every 3 months by his Endocrinologist who has taken the lead as his primary physician. Donato literally got his life back.

Michelle continues to fiercely advocate for everyone with symptoms of Auto-Brewery Syndrome. She is our educator in chief on the support group page, contacting every new member and offering help and her willingness to talk offline 24/7. With member input, she created a New Member Welcome document that includes a summary of nearly everything we know in our assembly. I can't count the number of doctors, hospitals, labs, and medical organizations she has contacted. Keep up your energy and good work, Michelle!

CHAPTER 12

DIAGNOSIS: IS IT REALLY AUTO-BREWERY SYNDROME?

Listen to your patient, he is telling you the diagnosis.

— *William Osler, Founder of Johns Hopkins Hospital*

THE NOSE KNOWS

Caregivers of patients with ABS report difficult-to-describe breath odors in the patients. Nearly all of us identify an unusual odor during a flare that is not typical of someone who has been drinking. Here are two descriptions from caregivers posted on the Facebook Support Page:

Julia: *B. has issues with breath during episodes...it's not an alcohol smell, more of a chemical smell. I used to think it was acetone but there was no acetone in his blood results, so I am just not sure.*

Sierra: *I work with essential oils, alcohols, etc. in my soap business as well as having spent years in research labs. I know what ethanol smells like compared to isopropyl alcohol (rubbing alcohol). R's breath changes with flares. Sometimes it's sweet, sometimes he smells like someone poured a bottle of vodka over him, and usually (mid or late flare) he starts smelling like metabolized alcohol (the standard hangover coming through the pores smell). But that is not a hard and fast rule.*

He rarely if ever smells like straight-out-of-the-bottle beer, vodka, or wine. He smells....different. And he doesn't smell like that 24/7. He literally might have a single exhaled breath that smells kind of boozy, which makes no sense if you know he hasn't been drinking. It smells like fermented fruit, sometimes like apples, occasionally like

*fermenting corn, and sometimes I can't give it a name. But none of those smells are exactly
the same as inhaling the smell from a bottle of regular ethanol.*

*Last night, while he was sleeping, he would exhale, and I felt like I was back in the
organic chemistry lab in college. His individual exhalations smelled like organic solvents. So, I
went looking for a way to describe it to someone who doesn't have a background in chem labs or
a few scientific degrees. Here's what I found. Not my words but written by a chemist on a blog:*

> Individually, [people with dysbiosis] tend to have distinctive
> odors. A good example is benzaldehyde - the smell of mara-
> schino cherries, and the reason they smell that way. I had a friend
> who refused to eat maraschinos - he called them 'benzaldehyde
> cherries.' Citral (the smell of lemon grass oil) and cinnamalde-
> hyde (the smell of cinnamon) and vanillin (the smell of vanilla)
> are all aldehydes. Acetaldehyde - which is halfway between eth-
> anol and acetic acid, smells sort of in between - sharp but not
> sour. A person can smell it in their own breath the morning after
> drinking too much vodka (along with acetic acid, too).[163]

MEDICAL BREATH TESTING

Doctors used their noses for centuries in detecting health issues. In the
fourth century BCE, Hippocrates instructed students to smell a patient's
breath to detect the sweetness of what we now call diabetes, the urine
smell of kidney failure, and the odor of fermented spirits as the cause of
drunken behavior.

In 1971, Linus Pauling and others authored a landmark paper identifying over 250 distinct substances in exhaled breath as measured by gas-liquid
partition chromatography.[164] Thus, began the race to include such testing for
diagnostic purposes.

---

163   Bassnotes. Aldehydes: What are they and what do they really smell like? http://www.basenotes.
net/threads/209281-Aldehydes-what-are-they-and-what-do-they-really-smell-like Retrieved 10-12-18

164   Pauling L, Robinson A, Teranish R, Cary P. (1971) Quantitative analysis of urine vapor and breath
by gas-liquid partition chromatography. *Proc Nat Acad Sci USA* 68(10):2374-2376

Today, modern gas chromatography and mass spectrometry (GC-MS) instruments enable us to analyze a complex sample depending on its chemical signature or mass -- the quantity of each chemical. We can identify more than 1000 unique substances in exhaled breath.[165]

Common examples of breath testing include a urea breath test to detect the overgrowth of *Helicobacter pylori* in peptic ulcer disease and exhaled nitric oxide that may signal airway inflammation in asthma and other conditions.

Breath tests for hydrogen and methane are non-invasive tests used frequently in differential diagnosis of gastrointestinal disorders such as carbohydrate malabsorption, small intestinal bacterial overgrowth (SIBO) and for measuring Oro-Cecal transit time (from mouth to cecum). Bacterial overgrowth produces hydrogen (H_2). Bacterial fermentation of leftover carbohydrates not absorbed in the small intestine generates methane (CH_4).[166]

These common breath tests are very important to a person suffering from ABS. Many of our ABS patients report flares when they eat food or drinks with artificial sweeteners and breath testing can detect malabsorption of artificial sweeteners. The doctors can determine if the symptoms of ABS overlap with other disorders such as food intolerances or SIBO. We might also look for associations between ABS and other conditions.

Here's an example of overlapping conditions: Andrea Lupascu and her colleagues at Catholic University of the Sacred Heart in Rome, Italy[167] revealed an association between Irritable Bowel Syndrome (IBS) and SIBO through a case control study. They recommended placebo controlled SIBO eradication studies to clarify the impact of SIBO on IBS.

---

165   Dweik R, Amann A. (2008) Exhaled breath analysis: the new frontier in medical testing. *J Breath Res* 2(3): https://doi.org/10.1088/1752-7163%2F2%2F3%2F030301

166   Rana S, Malik A. (2014) Breath tests and irritable bowel syndrome. *World J of Gastro* 20(24):7587-7601

167   Lupascu A, Gabrielli M, Lauritano E, et al. (2005) Hydrogen glucose breath test to detect small intestinal bacterial overgrowth: a prevalence case-control study in irritable bowel syndrome. *Alimen Pharm and Ther* 22:1157-1160. https://doi.org/10.1111/j.1365-2036.2005.02690.x

Breath testing is a non-invasive way to differentiate a diagnosis of IBS from other or overlapping diseases. Eleanora Nucera and others also from the Catholic University of the Sacred Heart in Rome, Italy[168] conducted a study of 98 patients with a diagnosis of IBS where those that had SIBO (as determined by breath tests) were treated with antibiotics and retested. They determined that eradication of SIBO normalizes sugar breath tests and therefore recommend those tests should be performed first to avoid a sugar malabsorption misdiagnosis.

The ABS community has much to learn from these studies and it would behoove researchers to include sufferers of ABS in similar clinical research.

· · · · · ·

Many of our ABS patients were tested with H_2 and CH_4 breath tests and the results generally came back negative unless there was a concomitant issue such as SIBO. As a precaution, patients with symptoms of ABS should request breath testing to rule out other GI health issues.

However, H_2 breath testing can also be used for diagnosing rapid or slow transit time of food through the small intestine.[169] I believe these particular tests are important for anyone who has symptoms of ABS and here is why: other confirmed cases of ABS have been reported in people with Short Bowel Syndrome, people with dilatation, reverse peristalsis, and retention of food or contrast medium. You want to know if you have any underlying condition.

Jejunoileal bypass surgery for medically complicated obesity is where the jejunum or near-beginning of the small intestine and the ileum or end of the small intestine is joined, removing what's in between. Over one-third of patients who had this surgery have elevated concentrations of blood ethanol

---

168   Nucera G, Gabrielli M, Lupascu A, et al. (2005) Abnormal breath tests to lactose, fructose and sorbitol in irritable bowel syndrome may be explained by small intestinal bacterial overgrowth. *Alimen Pharm and Ther* 21:1391-1395. https://doi.org/10.1111/j.1365-2036.2005.02493.x

169   Rana S, Malik A. (2014) Hydrogen breath tests in gastrointestinal diseases. *Ind J Clin Biochem* 29(4):398–405. DOI 10.1007/s12291-014-0426-4

after surgery.[170] Many of our ABS patients report alternating between constipation and diarrhea so perhaps there is a link to transit time, overgrowth of yeast, and endogenous ethanol production.

MEASURING ETHANOL AND HOW IT RELATES TO ABS

Even though exhaled acetone and ethanol could be mechanically detected in breath as early as the mid-1800s, the use of our noses continued well into the 20th century because testing was expensive, laborious, and unreliable.

Dr. Francis Edmond Anstie was the first to measure ethanol, also known as ethyl alcohol, or more commonly alcohol. He lived in London in the 1860s and developed a reagent to quantify alcohol in urine.[171] Building on Anstie's work, a young Swede, Erik Widmark, pioneered the blood measurement of alcohol in 1922.[172] And in 1927, American Dr. Emil Bogen was the first to demonstrate that breath samples could correlate to a blood alcohol level.[173]

The precursor to the current day breathalyzer was a device called a "drunkometer" invented by Rolla Harger at Indiana University in the 1930s. It was a portable device with a rubber balloon attached to a tube filled with a weak solution of potassium permanganate in sulfuric acid. If a person had been drinking and blew into the tube, the solution changed from clear to purple with a darker color indicating higher alcohol levels.[174]

I wonder how Dr. Harger could take the measurement of alcohol seriously with something called a drunkometer! Plus, as seen in Image 8, it looks quite humorous as well.

---

170   Nair S, Cope K, Terrence R, Diehl A. (2001) Obesity and female gender increase breath ethanol concentrations: Potential implications for the pathogenesis of nonalcoholic steatohepatitis. *The Amer J Gastro* 96(4):1200-1204

171   Baldwin A. (1977) Anstie's alcohol limit. *Amer J Public Health* 67(7):679-681

172   Jones A. (2009) Erik MP Widmark - Bridged the Gap Between Forensic Toxicology and Alcohol and Traffic Safety Research. *Blutalcohol*

173   Bogen E. (1927) The diagnosis of drunkenness: A quantitative study of acute alcoholic intoxication. *California and Western Medicine* 26(6):778-779

174   McGill. (2018). Before the Breathalyzer, there was the Drunkometer. https://www.mcgill.ca/oss/article/did-you-know-history/breathalyzer-there-was-drunkometer

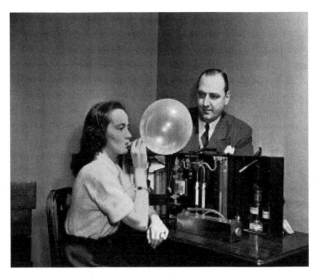

Image 8: Photo taken on March 28, 1950 (AP/Carl Nesensohn)
License: <u>CC by: Attribution</u>

But the device was simple, easy to use and fairly reliable; experiments demonstrated that illness and food eaten did not affect the results. With the drunkometer able to accompany police officers in a small suitcase, the authorities soon realized just how many people were driving drunk.

In the1950s, the breathalyzer replaced the drunkometer. Robert Borkenstein, another Indiana University professor, invented the new device for use in the field. The breathalyzer is a much smaller and more sophisticated device that uses infrared spectroscopy to measure breath alcohol levels (BrAC). It is the current law enforcement standard for screening.[175] Most breathalyzers now may rely on either infrared or fuel cell technologies.[176]

Modern laboratories in the United States currently use an array of sophisticated equipment to determine blood alcohol levels (BAC) through processes such as gas chromatography, enzymatic oxidation, chemical

175 Blood Alcohol Concentration, Measures of. *Encyclopedia of Drugs, Alcohol, and Addictive Behavior*. 23 Jul. 2018 <u>http://www.encyclopedia.com</u>

176 Morey T, Booth M, Prather R, et al. (2011). Measurement of ethanol in gaseous breath using a miniature gas chromatograph. *J Anal Toxicol* 35(3):134-142

oxidation (enzyme assays) and osmometry. The 260,000 labs in the U.S. are regulated through the Clinical Laboratory Improvement Amendments (CLIA)[177] and are standardized and reliable.

It is important to stress there are two types of *blood* ethanol tests; one is a routine clinical analysis (BAC) and the other is a legal blood alcohol test (LBAT). Headspace gas chromatography for LBAT is "the current forensic gold standard" for ethanol analysis.[178]

· · · · · ·

Remember, I said earlier that in the U.S. we measure blood alcohol concentration (BAC) in mg/dL and breath alcohol concentrations (BrAC) in mg%. The two are often both called BAC, so it can be confusing. For example, a BAC of 314 mg/dL would correspond to a BrAC of 0.31mg% usually shortened to 0.31% or .31. Several other countries use mg/ml or mg/L so don't get muddled – ask for the units of measurement if you are uncertain.

To be precise, blood and breath measures of alcohol do not always agree. The Encyclopedia of Drugs, Alcohol and Addiction states:

> …breath-ethanol analyzers were calibrated in such a way that the readout was obtained directly in terms of the *presumed* BAC [emphasis mine]. In the United States and elsewhere, a blood/ breath factor of 2,100:1 was approved for legal purposes with the understanding that this gives a margin of safety (about 10%) to the accused. Indeed, more recent research suggests that the blood/breath factor should be 2,300:1 for closer agreement between direct BAC and the result derived from BrAC.[179]

---

177   Centers for Medicare and Medicaid Services. https://www.cms.gov/Regulations-and-Guidance/ Legislation/CLIA/index.html?redirect=/CLIA

178   Platteborze P, Willhelms K. (2017) Legal blood alcohol testing in the U.S. Military. *Military Medicine* 182:e1558-e1561. IP: 202.177.173.189

179   Blood Alcohol Concentration, Measures of. *Encyclopedia of Drugs, Alcohol, and Addictive Behavior* 23 Jul. 2018 http://www.encyclopedia.com

BAC and BrAC are usually highly correlated, and the levels as well as the metabolism of alcohol in the body can be monitored with either method; however, BrAC measurements are more prone to physiological variations such as body and breath temperature, pulmonary function, and pattern of breathing prior to exhalation.[180] This is why when someone is arrested on suspicion of DUI, they can and should request a blood draw to verify or refute the breathalyzer reading. Typically, a court would require a legal blood alcohol test (LBAT) anyway.

Nanocomposite technology is the future of BrAC measurement. Within the last decade, Dr. Timothy Morey and eight of his collaborators from the University of Florida School of Medicine[181] "designed and built a new generation of a breath-based ethanol detection device based on miniature gas chromatography (mGC) with a metal oxide sensor for real-time, point-of-need detection of ethanol concentrations" (p.134). Soon, the new device will enable the BrAC to be as accurate as the BAC.

In summary, there is a difference in the way our common breathalyzers work compared to blood measurements and even forensic technology. We've had several patients who detect a BrAC that does not match the BAC from the hospital laboratory. You need to be aware of the discrepancies. BrAC is a great screening device, but for medical diagnosis or forensic purposes, you will need a BAC or LBAT.

DIAGNOSING ABS

The most common question I get about ABS is "How do you know if you have Auto-Brewery?" I'll discuss the major elements of diagnosis here and treatment in Chapter 16, but I also put together a bulleted list in Appendix B for quick reference.

---

180   Lenos J. (2016) Improved environmental operation of alcohol breathalyzers with functionalized graphene nanocomposite membranes *UWSpace* http://hdl.handle.net/10012/10800

181   Morey T, Booth M, Prather R, et al. (2011) Measurement of ethanol in gaseous breath using a miniature gas chromatograph. *J Anal Toxicol* 35(3):134-142

First, get a journal or logbook where you can record times throughout each day – one day per page is a good format. Religiously keep track of every bite of food you eat and every sip you drink; really everything you put in your mouth. Don't forget to record mints, gum, smoking and dipping activities. Add a column to track activity such as work, leisure, exercise, sports, and sleep. In the next column document your mood or feelings during the activity (stressed, relaxed, worried, etc.)

Another important column in your logbook should include any symptoms you experience, like stupor, drunkenness, slurred words, dilated pupils, foul or strange breath. If you have a partner or family member who can help with the recording, even better, since you may not even be aware of many of these symptoms. Within a week or two you should see patterns emerge.

The best way to know if you are fermenting ethanol is to buy a Department of Transportation (DOT) approved breathalyzer and test your breath alcohol concentration (BrAC) when you feel symptomatic. You can purchase a high-quality breathalyzer for around $100. There are cheaper models available, but they are not as accurate, so I recommend getting the higher end model. Be sure to read the directions and follow them in order to get a correct reading. Most machines have a calibration method and require at least a 30-minute wait after eating or drinking to test.

Important: if you've been drinking, an elevated level doesn't count toward proving ABS. If you haven't had anything to drink, and your BrAC is elevated to anything above 0.00, this is a strong indicator that your gut has a problem. If you've had very little to drink and your BrAC is unusually high, this may also be an indicator, but it confuses the issue.

If you discover elevated alcohol levels, it is important to document your BrAC throughout the day along with that ever-important activity and symptom journal or logbook. This information is essential when you approach a healthcare provider for diagnosis and treatment.

Most diagnoses have been made through a thorough history with detailed symptoms documented by a patient journal. Allow a loved one to help you record your activities, food, and symptoms since you may not recognize or remember them when you are flaring or after.

Some of our caregivers recommend you approach a doctor with the detailed logbook without mentioning ABS just to get a foot in the door. Find an open-minded Gastrointestinal (GI) or Infectious Disease doctor who will conduct breath testing to rule out other diseases, or to zero in on diseases that may mimic, overlap, or confuse the ABS diagnosis. The website lists the doctors we know of that currently treat ABS: www.autobrewery.info.

Be aware that existing conditions such as diabetes or liver problems can impact the diagnosis of ABS. Patients with type II diabetes mellitus (DM) or liver cirrhosis (LC) had higher endogenous ethanol (EnEth) levels than a control group without the disease. But the researchers found the highest EnEth levels in a fourth group of patients with both type II DM and LC where the BAC increases reached 22.3 mg/dL.[182,183] This is one of many reasons it's important to tell your doctor your complete health history.

••••••

All of our ABS patients report dietary triggers, but they aren't 100% consistent, even within a single patient's experience. In other words, some people have episodes, or flares within two hours of a trigger, others up to 24 to 48 hours later, and not always with the same foods. Some flare with glucose but others only with high fructose corn syrup (HFCS) -- which may be influenced by other factors such as additional food eaten prior to, or at the same time.

Bizarrely, our patients report some of their worst flares in response to environmental toxins aside from food. For example, snuff, dip, or chewing tobacco have many suspicious ingredients and cause very serious flares in many patients with ABS (see Appendix A). We are not sure why these

---

182   Simic M, Ajdukovic N, Veselinovic I., et al. (2012) Endogenous ethanol production in patients with diabetes mellitus as a medicolegal problem. *For Sci Intl* 216:97-100

183   Hafez E, Hamad M, Fouad M, Abdel-Lateff A. (2017) Auto-Brewery Syndrome: Ethanol pseudo-toxicity in diabetic and hepatic patients. *Human Exp Tox* 36(5):445-450. https://doi. org/10.1177/0960327116661400

substances would trigger fermentation, but we have many documented episodes directly tied to these toxins.

Even stranger, many ABS patients report flares in response to chemical exposure such as solvents, glues, paint thinners, and other fumes. So, it's not just what they put in their mouths, it's the world around us; the whole environment contains hazards that can trigger flares of gut fermentation in people with yeast overgrowth. Many in the support community believe environmental toxins are very much connected to ABS (see Appendix A).

Sarah: *My husband's first symptoms with auto-brewery syndrome started after he used a very strong solvent-based sealant on a wood floor. That night he developed intoxication symptoms although we did not know what it was at the time. I made him go to a doctor to discuss what had happened and [the doctor] just said it was a reaction and T. should be careful with solvents and paints in the future. He did not use the sealant anymore but continued having episodes.*

Before being diagnosed with ABS, Joe was using a solvent to remove old vinyl tile flooring in our garage. He started around 9:00 a.m. and by 10:00 a.m. was totally incapacitated by the fumes. He lost coordination, couldn't talk and had to go to bed. When the same thing happened the next day, I made him stop and I finished the job of removing the tiles. I thought he was having a reaction to the solvent, but in retrospect, I believe it triggered his fermentation and he was drunk.

And there are other chemical toxins in our air that possibly contribute to ABS.

Dave (ABS patient): *My nephew and I were discussing engine combustion in cold ambient temperatures and the addition of ethanol in gasoline. I stated that my ABS condition got worse in the winter. We've had 10% ethanol in regular gas for several years here in Ontario and our government is pushing for 20% to meet carbon emissions reduction, which really concerns me.*

Research confirms that ethanol and acetaldehyde emissions are up to 30% higher in the cold weather than in summer from vehicles burning ethanol blends. Cold air prevents the pollutants from rising into the atmosphere by way of convection.[184] Remember that acetaldehyde is an intermediary in alcohol metabolism and both ethanol and acetaldehyde are toxic to humans. Perhaps inhaled ethanol and acetaldehyde trigger gut fermentation and a flare in patients with yeast overgrowth.

STRESS

S tress is another major trigger for ABS flares. A patient may not necessarily feel stressed, but stress at work or in traffic can provoke a flare. Even the stress of skipping a meal or strenuous yard work can spark an episode. Feelings of stress are important to capture in the logbook. Stress is a huge factor in all our lives – so much so that we may be inclined to dismiss it as a health issue because we all experience stress to some degree and must cope with stressful days and events.

But let's remember that stress is on a spectrum from very low stress all the way to debilitating stress to the point of anxiety, panic attacks, and even Post Traumatic Stress Disorder (PTSD). Many people experience levels of stress that most of us can only imagine and that can be a point of shame. I'll talk more about stress and stress management in the treatment chapter.

Many of our patients also believe there may be a genetic link for ABS and are paying to have DNA analyses with health profiles done; however, commercial companies are not set up to determine genetic errors, such as in enzyme production, the way researchers can. We need researchers to pursue some of these leads.

Dr. Kanodia and I discovered in our research that patients with ABS (N=28) have significant differences compared to people without ABS (N=18). Thirteen of the 60 lifestyle, diet and health history questions showed statistical significance between those with and without ABS.[185]

---

184   Suarez-Bertoa R, Zardini A, Kueken H, Astorga C. (2015) Impact of ethanol containing gasoline blends on emissions from a fex-fuel vehicle tested over the Worldwide Harmonized Light duty Text Cycle (WLTC). *Fuel* 143:173-182. http://dx.doi.org/10.1016/j.fuel.2014.10.076

185   Cordell B, Kanodia A, Miller G. (2019) Case control research study on Auto-Brewery Syndrome. *Global Advances in Health and Medicine* 8:1-7. https://doi.org/10.1177/2164956119837566

In summary, the hallmarks of ABS are 1) the endogenous production of alcohol and 2) gut dysbiosis with an overgrowth of yeast. But there are many other elements going on here such as triggers, sensitivities and toxins. Additional research is needed because we have a long way to go to understand other coinciding and underlying factors. There are many pieces to the puzzle.

PROVING THE DIAGNOSIS

If you are trying to prove you have ABS to someone else, like law enforcement, your family, or a dis-believing healthcare provider, that may be considerably harder. A primary provider (M.D., Nurse Practitioner, DO, etc.) would need to admit you to a hospital or other controlled environment for a 24-hour observation without access to alcohol. Then they (and you) try to recreate the triggers that cause the drunkenness by using a glucose challenge or a high carbohydrate diet (sugar, pasta, corn, or your particular triggers).

You should be prepared for the possibility that you may not flare during the observation. Not all triggers can be reproduced in a hospital such as solvents, smoking, and specific stressors. For example, stress from physical labor is difficult to replicate in a hospital, although hospitalization itself is a stressor.

Some people report delayed responses where episodes or flares happen up to two days later, so a flare may or may not happen within a monitored 24-hour hospital stay. We may need to get more creative with out-patient monitoring. The main element is assuring the patient has no access to alcohol.

One patient's attorney, Joseph Marusak, hired two nurses and a physician's assistant to follow his client around 24/7 to ensure she did not ingest alcohol. They stayed with her until she registered an elevated blood alcohol level. Her defense was effective, and the DWI charge was dismissed.[186] You'll hear more about this case in the chapter on Legal Issues.

---

186   CNN. (2016). Woman claims her body brews alcohol: has DUI charge dismissed. https://www.cnn.com/2015/12/31/health/auto-brewery-syndrome-dui-womans-body-brews-own-alcohol/index.html

While in the hospital or controlled environment, a breathalyzer may be used for screening, and blood would be drawn for BAC every few hours to corroborate any rise in breath alcohol by the breathalyzer. Glucose levels should be tested as well, especially if you are a diabetic. But even without diabetes many people with ABS have transient blood sugar problems, either elevated blood sugar, or hypoglycemia so checking blood glucose is still important.

Prior to the observation, the primary provider will conduct a detailed history including your logbook and send stool samples for yeast cultures and DNA identification. Not all stool samples come back positive for yeast and a gastroenterologist should do a complete workup, which may include colonoscopy and esophagogastroduodenoscopy (EGD) - there's one of those medical words I love! The additional samples from these tests are for yeast DNA identification from other locations along the GI tract.

One hundred percent of our patients diagnosed with ABS, as well as all the published cases, grew positive yeast cultures from a sample taken somewhere in the intestines. Lab testing is an important aspect of diagnosis to determine the type of yeast that is overgrowing and causing the fermentation of ethanol. Our doctors use Quest, Genova, and other laboratories for DNA testing of yeast.

Gordon: *We had a doctor that utilized Genova labs in the past. They have a good bacterial DNA database and the most complete (at the time, 2013) fungal DNA database. Dr. L. was able to make some substantial recommendations based on their testing data in my case.*

SYMPTOMS THAT MAY ACCOMPANY ABS

Symptoms of common yeast overgrowth include itchy, flaky skin, toe fungus, vaginal or jock itch, athlete's foot, dandruff, and fatigue, and may or may not occur along with ABS. People with ABS might have all, some, or none of these symptoms.

It makes sense that a disturbed microbiome might allow yeast to grow somewhere on the skin as well as the gut. But people with any of these symptoms of yeast infection may not ever develop ABS and people with ABS may not have skin yeast infections.

Many people with ABS experience gastric upset such as nausea, vomiting, bloating, belching, and flatulence. ABS has been strongly correlated with leaky gut syndrome, food sensitivities, SIBO, and *Helicobacter pylori*.

H. pylori is one of those bacteria found in over 50% of humans and we know it's an important regulatory species passed from mother to child generally for life. What we are not sure of yet is whether it's a commensal, a pathogen, or a protector.[187] It may play all three roles depending on the host and the environment.

Gastroesophageal reflux disease or GERD may be diagnosed in a patient long before ABS. If patients have some of these collateral conditions they may confound, confuse, or make the ABS diagnosis more challenging and the management more difficult.

Our patients report varying degrees of severity of symptoms. Some patients may only flare intermittently and others several times a day. Some patients rarely vomit while others experience near constant nausea and vomiting. This may be due to the virulent nature of the yeast or the amount of overgrowth. It may also be due to the lack of homeostasis with other gut microbes.

The auto-brewery support group discussed some of the more unusual symptoms of ABS and their triggers and we've put together a chart to help others and aid in research. Appendix A lists many of the symptoms with triggers, underlying chemistry or biochemistry, and possible links. Our citizen scientists continue to explore links and possible avenues of research to fill in the blanks of our medical scotoma.

---

187   Whalen M, Massidda O. (2015) Helicobacter pylori: enemy, commensal or sometimes, friend? *J Infect Dev Countries* 9:674-678. DOI: https://doi.org/10.3855/jidc.7186

CHAPTER 13 🪱

THE CALL TO ACTION

The freedom of patient speech is necessary if the doctor is to get clues about the medical enigma before him. If the patient is inhibited, or cut off prematurely, or constrained into one path of discussion, then the doctor may not be told something vital. Observers have noted that, on average, physicians interrupt patients within eighteen seconds of when they begin telling their story.

— Jerome Groopman, MD, Author for the New Yorker

THE DANGERS OF MISDIAGNOSIS

One of the scariest outcomes of any patient-provider encounter is misdiagnosis. Even before the realization that a person is drunk, as a matter of due diligence a concerned doctor may look for causes of the patient's reported symptoms: weakness, slurred words, lack of coordination, sleep apnea, snoring, sudden loss of consciousness, or seizures.

Many ABS patients went to their primary doctor early on to try and figure out why they felt fatigued and slurred their words. Their doctors would perform blood tests, A1C levels, glucose challenges, neurological exams, CAT scans, gastro-endoscopies, colonoscopies, and many other tests that often revealed nothing.

Barbara Ehrenreich, in her recent book, *Natural Causes,* states what many of us already know: "In the laboratory-centered environment, the patient's words – his or her medical history and reported symptoms – count for less than the objective data that instruments can collect."[188]

ABS patients report feeling fine in terms of cognitive function except when they have a flare, yet doctors still want to conduct expensive, time-intensive neurological tests because they trust the EEG and the CAT scan over patient accounts. These same doctors are often surprised when all 'objective tests' come back normal.

To be fair, many people have symptoms related to ABS that can easily be mistaken for something else. This goes back to our horses-not-zebras principle. For example, the blood sugar levels often soar or dip precipitously when a person with ABS flares and so, some patients are misdiagnosed with low blood sugar (hypoglycemia) or Type II or Type I diabetes.

Once the ABS is under control, the blood sugar issues often abate as well. Stacey's story is a good example; she was diagnosed with Type I diabetes before she realized she had ABS. Once she was treated for her ABS, she no longer needed insulin. Years later, Stacey progressed from pre-diabetic to Type II and then Type I diabetes and there may be a connection with ABS since her wild blood sugar swings occurred during flares. Perhaps ABS stresses the pancreas.

Some of our patients underwent neurological workups to rule out stroke, ischemia, and other possible causes of their symptoms. They didn't understand what was happening because they hadn't been drinking. ABS is known to deplete certain minerals such as B vitamins, zinc, and magnesium[189] and consequently, patients, again like Stacey, may be misdiagnosed with Gitelman Syndrome, kidney disfunction, or mineral deficiency.

Our patients report being misdiagnosed with:

- Gitelman's Syndrome or Bartter's Syndrome

- Depression

---

188   Ehrenreich B. (2018) *Natural Causes* New York:12

189   Eaton K, McLaren H, Hunnisett A, Harris M. (2004) Abnormal gut fermentation: Laboratory studies reveal deficiency of B vitamins, zinc, and magnesium. *J Nutr & Envir Med* 14(2):115-120

- Type I or II Diabetes

- Hypoglycemia

- Dementia

- Neurological problems of unknown origin

- Seizure Disorders

- Sleep Deprivation due to Sleep Apnea

- Hypochondriac

- Severe alcoholism accompanied by denial

Compounding the difficulty of an accurate diagnosis is the wait time for specialists' appointments. Many patients cannot get an appointment sooner than six weeks or even three months! How hard is it for a doctor to order a 24-hour hospital observation to witness a flare with his or her own eyes? A 24-hour observation could also provide the prized objective lab results.

PLEASE LISTEN TO US

Those of us in the auto-brewery support community deeply value the handful of primary providers who have listened to us with an open mind and a compassionate heart. We know these care providers like Dr. McCarthy, Dr. Kanodia, Dr. Wick, Dr. Jesse and others saved the lives of our ABS patients.

Sadly, this is not the norm. Most of us interacted with multiple providers who shunned us before we found the one outlier who listened. How do you trust a doctor, who has the power to make such important decisions, when he or she doesn't believe you? It instantly becomes a fundamentally dysfunctional relationship.

Every single ABS patient or caregiver who has called or emailed me recounts harrowing stories of rebuke. We were shamed and blamed and turned away. I was told "it's impossible for the body to produce alcohol," and Joe "must be a closet alcoholic," when I was a Ph.D. nurse researcher standing right there with the literature in my hand.

Stacey's doctor told Larry that Stacey "must be hiding alcohol," and then she was misdiagnosed first with diabetes and then with Gitelman's syndrome. Meanwhile, she regularly felt like she was about to die.

Donato was hospitalized 22 times before Michelle demanded to find a doctor who would diagnose and treat him. Nick and Karen were told that Nick was "just an alcoholic" and Ray and Sierra, who you will read about in Chapters 15 and 16, are informed by a judge and prosecutor that Auto-Brewery Syndrome does not exist, so "Ray must be drinking and lying."

I mentioned shame in the chapter on alcoholism, and ABS is burdened with that same shame that somehow patients and families are lying or in denial. There are variations on the theme but all families with ABS have experienced at the very least, embarrassment by the statements of an ignorant or insensitive doctor, and at the worst, humiliation, harassment, and accusations by a total ass of a doctor. It is a disease, people!

••••••

I don't mean to be unsympathetic to doctors; you worked hard to get where you are, and I believe most of you started off with the best of intentions. Think back to the beginning of your medical training and the dreams you had of helping people and caring for the vulnerable sick. What happened to the young scientist who went to medical school because you loved the investigative work of diagnosis and wanted to truly help people?

Unfortunately, the medical system socializes medical interns as free-of-charge employees, and forces residents to work grueling 24-hour shifts. You had little time off, even less time to sleep, and were paid next to nothing for your services.

Many nights on the late shift as a nurse I had to wake up the bleary-eyed resident on call and hear him give a crazy order I then had to question. One night, I called a resident for a patient's heart rate of 50 and he told me to administer digoxin, a medication that slows the heart rate. I refused the order, but the resident argued with me, so I called the Chief Resident to override the order. I believe the resident was so exhausted, his brain wasn't working correctly.

Part of the problem is that you start off with a "scientist brain" wanting to search, discover, and learn. Then the massive education and training you engage in promote an "expert brain" that tells you you've learned everything you need to know to be a great doctor. These two brains may conflict with one another.

This same medical-industrial complex tries to convince new doctors that you have sacrificed so much to achieve the coveted medical degree with board certifications that you deserve every penny you can charge and can finally live a well-deserved life of luxury. There are many well-known books about how this system of medical education came to be that show altruism and compassion have a hard time surviving this harsh socialization.

Doctors who are emotionally sensitive to their patients are more likely to experience exhaustion, burnout, and stress-related illness.[190] No wonder you doctors build up emotional defenses to protect yourselves. I only want to encourage you to look at your behavior toward patients and family members. I challenge you to listen to us with an open mind and maintain, or regain, your scientific rigor and human compassion.

Many of our patients and caregivers turn to primary health professionals such as doctors of osteopathy (DOs), Physician Assistants (PAs), and Nurse Practitioners (NPs and DNPs) when they are turned away by conventional physicians. The philosophical underpinnings of training these pros are quite different from conventional medicine.

For example, the theory of nursing is built on a process, a system, or a philosophy of caring, holism, patient dignity and patient autonomy. Even though nurse practitioners can diagnose medical ailments and prescribe

---

190   Amoafo E, Hanbali N, Patel A, Singh P. (2015) What are the significant factors associated with burnout in doctors? *Occupational Medicine* 65(2):117-121. http://doi.org/10.1093/occmed/kqu144

medications, they have first been trained to diagnose human and holistic needs of body, mind, and spirit.

Whatever your background and training, if you are a first-line provider, you need equal parts of scientific inquiry, diagnostic skill, and caring. I know you all have tight schedules and you want to help as many people as possible as efficiently as possible, but please remember your initial investigative mind. Remember the Hippocratic oath to first "do no harm", so please, no shaming. And most importantly – LISTEN TO YOUR PATIENTS with an open mind - don't assume everyone who is drunk is lying.

CHAPTER 14

THE INVISIBLE DISEASE: RAY (PATIENT) AND SIERRA (RAY'S WIFE)

> *Today we fight. Tomorrow we fight. The day after, we fight. And if this disease plans on whipping us, it better bring a lunch, 'cause it's gonna have a long day doing it.*
>
> — *Jim Beaver, Life's That Way*

Sierra contacted me in January of 2017. She joined our confidential support group but had already started her own Facebook support page. She is a key citizen scientist who says, *"I started this page to show what REALLY happens when life happens, and you're suddenly knocked flat on your ass by health issues from ABS."*

Sierra rarely leaves Ray's side now but bought him a GPS tracker for those scarce times when they must be apart. Sierra and Ray's story is a tragic tale of how disruptive ABS can be to people's lives, livelihoods, and finances. They aren't the only ones.

Ray is a former U.S. Army paratrooper from Eugene, OR who overturned a vehicle carrying 11,000 salmon "under the influence" in December 2014. Ray doesn't drink, but he realized in retrospect he'd been suffering from drunken-like attacks a year before the accident. He was diagnosed with ABS in August 2015. He lost that truck driving job after a long fight with the company over the medical diagnosis and his legal battle continues to this day.

Like most ABS patients, Ray had a hard time finding a doctor in Oregon who recognized the syndrome and because of his legal struggles, Ray is not allowed to leave the state for treatment. Ray's condition is also chronic, as he has not responded to the usual treatments and continues even now to experience flares.

Sierra: *Ray is an avid outdoorsman, having learned to fish before he could walk. He was tying his own flies for fly-fishing for trout in tiny mountain streams by age eleven. Most content in the middle of nowhere, miles from a paved road or civilization, he finds quiet inside when it is peaceful outside and he's knee-deep in flowing water.*

He served his country as a mortar team squad leader (AKA grunt) in the 82nd Airborne – Italy (1987 – 1990) and then as a Senior Scout Observer in the Long-Range Surveillance Detachment (Airborne) –Iraq, Kuwait, Bahrain, Qatar, and Saudi Arabia (1990 – 1991). Ray was an exemplary employee for Oregon Department of Fish & Wildlife from 2004 to 2016, when he was fired because of his unknown medical condition that caused an accident in 2014.

I am a 5th generation Texan who refuses to quit (especially when I know I'm right). I grew up sitting in one place just watching nature as it went about its business of living. What I couldn't see in nature, I researched in books. I knew I wanted to be a field biologist back in high school. I now have a B.S. in Marine Biology from Texas A&M University (1999) and an M.S. in Fisheries Science from Oregon State University (2013).

Ray and I met in 2000 in San Diego, California while I was on a post-college adventure and Ray was trying to go back to school with his GI Bill benefits. We married in 2006 and have one very fuzzy, 13-year-old, deaf kitty named Doppler.

I've spent my entire life navigating the complexities of the medical industry. Being a rare disease (cancer) survivor myself for 40 years, I've been helping Ray come to terms with his medical realities as they appear.

Ray: *This is not who I am. This is not who I want to be.*

Sierra: *It's easier to just shut down and not try to interact than it is to explain what each day's challenge has been. This disease robs him of his independence, his coordination, his beautiful sense of humor, and his ability to function in normal society.*

......

S ierra: *After his accident, Ray was referred from doctor to doctor, and finally to the ABS expert in Ohio, Dr. Anup Kanodia. Ray has also been under the care of the US Veterans Administration, located in Roseburg, Oregon, whose Primary Care Physician and Gastro-Intestinal Specialist acknowledge and treat him for ABS.*

He works at that same facility through the Work Therapy program, where they monitor his progress with ABS in a working environment, to determine how a person dealing with a life-long affliction such as ABS fits into what could be considered a normal working environment.

Ray: *After the long and expensive summer that led to the diagnosis of ABS, I was able to recount events and behaviors prior to the accident and recognize that there were symptoms of the disease earlier in that year. Unfortunately, I had no way of knowing what was going on at the time, particularly about a disease that I had no idea even existed.*

Looking back at that period in 2014 prior to the accident, I realize that my fatigue, high blood pressure, intestinal distress, lack of appetite, poor eating habits, and forgetfulness coincided with the onset of ABS. I knew prior to the accident that something was off with my health, but I did not know exactly what.

I had obtained a new PCP [primary care provider] *locally and had in fact been in his office the day before the accident and had an extensive panel of blood draws at his request.*

Aside from the obvious medical and legal issues that affect me directly, the worst part of the ordeal is what this has done to Sierra. She doesn't have ABS, but her life is completely immersed in it, nonetheless. Financially, emotionally, and physically, this has upended her life as a caregiver and spouse, and the disease offers no distinction in this regard between her or me.

Sierra: *3-19-17: Ray started a 2-week Diflucan prescription last week. We'll keep you posted. He is still on the original restricted diet plan and will not be deviating from it.*

9-8-17: Back at the ER: I don't have an explanation, but Ray blew a BAC of 0.461 after a 4-hour nap upstairs. He was almost nonverbal and was repeating "something's wrong." He couldn't walk well and barely made it to the car. [He is] *Very confused, asked where we were going 4 times in 45 minutes. And now he's reading at .29* [the average man would have to have 16 drinks to register this high].

I don't know if the BAC meter is freaking out at higher levels or what. The symptoms are much worse, so something is happening. I have no explanation for how the levels can drop so quickly otherwise. This sucks.

10-31-2017: Another appeal: I find myself at a loss of what to say. The entire legal appeal lasted 30 minutes. It was only the oral arguments after months of written briefs submitted by both Ray's lawyer and the State's lawyer. Highly anticlimactic given the almost three years we've been waiting for a decision. We won't know anything until the Appeals court issues a decision. In our case, longer is better because it usually means the judges are drafting some sort of decision — which deviates from the existing law. So, the longer it takes, theoretically the better for us.

In the meantime, we are still taking each day as it comes. Ray is still flaring and staying at BAC levels above .20+ for hours on end. The last one he hit .20+ on Friday night, woke up in the .20s on Saturday, and stayed in the .20s until early Sunday morning.

11-27-2017: We lost the appeal. Now it goes to the State Supreme court in Oregon who does not have to take the case. It will be months before we find out if they will even hear the case. Either way, we have to file for bankruptcy and move towards selling our farm and home.

······

S ierra: *I've been asked how we are paying for all the legal and medical expenses? Well, we literally don't have money for next month's mortgage payment, or the $4,000 dollars required by the appeal lawyer. If we can't raise the funds to continue (and win) the appeal process, Ray will owe $485k until he dies, and we lose the house, the farm, and everything we've worked toward over seventeen years together. Restitution for his "criminal" actions cannot ever be forgiven, even under bankruptcy.*

Ray hasn't worked for ODFW since the accident on December 30, 2014. After the accident, he was told by ODFW to not come back into the office until "the criminal issue" was resolved. He used up his accrued vacation and sick leave very quickly. He wasn't allowed to return to work at ODFW ever again. He was formally fired April 2016, three months after the trial ended.

"It's just money…, right?" Every dollar spent on Ray's medical and legal issues has come from me since January 2015. A combination of unexpected inheritance, retirement, savings, and meager paychecks have all been exhausted. Generous GoFundMe donations contributed more than $7,500 USD. It helped immensely with morale but didn't last very long when I had to write several checks in excess of $10,000 each to keep the legal fight moving forward (while also seeking medical treatment for Ray's ABS). We keep fighting.

••••••

Throughout the early months of 2018, Ray continued to flare every few days. It was like a roller coaster for him with spikes and dips in his BAC. He seemed very debilitated, barely able to dress himself. Sometimes he could not go to his part-time job at the VA. Ray and Sierra were trying every dietary, supplemental, and integrative therapy they could think of, but still he flared. Here are examples from Sierra's support group Facebook posts of their ongoing tribulations.

6-8-2018: We're here. It's the busiest time of year for our little farm so Ray is working outside clearing brush and weed-whacking while I'm trying to get the fruits and veggies set up for the growing season. We're basically running from sunup to sundown.

On the medical side, Ray just had a visit with Dr. Kanodia and it's time to do more testing to figure out which species of yeast and bacteria might be causing his flares. While the test methods are pretty straightforward (stool, blood, saliva), none of the tests are covered under his VA treatment - because there is no standard treatment or drug regimen for this obscure disease and NONE of it is covered under copays.

So, here's to another mortgage payment going out the door to doctors - for a disease that people think is a joke. I guarantee you; we are not laughing in this house.

6-10-2018: He started flaring yesterday because he overexerted himself putting fencing up that we need on our farm.

Ray: *The actual times of positive BAC are difficult, but not the sole medical issue presented by ABS. The recovery time after a BAC spike, or "flare," is wrought with extremely irritable bowel issues, dehydration, headache, disrupted sleep, and lack of energy, just to name a few symptoms. Even though I haven't consumed alcohol in the traditional way, my body simply doesn't care that it has been produced endogenously.*

My body's only concern is processing and functioning the best way it knows how under the circumstances. The same is often true even when there is no measurable BAC. My appetite can still be off, my sleep is often disrupted or prolonged, my blood pressure and pulse can fluctuate.

• • • • • •

S ierra: Lots of people live with rare, invisible diseases. You pass by them every day never seeing their illness because they're doing their best to hide it and look "normal." I've done that successfully for 40 years as a survivor of childhood cancer. Ray doesn't get that chance.

He gets judged, mocked, and treated with disrespect because people assume he's just another drunk. I can't tell you how angry that makes me as his wife. He is not a criminal, and he deserves the same legal treatment that undiagnosed diabetics and epileptics get when their disease reveals itself during a vehicle accident.

Here's hoping we can get these bad guys identified so they can be eradicated. While not cheap, this is the 3rd or 4th time since Ray's original diagnosis that we have done this test. Each test offers a snapshot count of the creatures living in Ray's intestines. *crosses fingers, toes, and legs*

POSTSCRIPT:

S ierra and Ray are grateful for the love and support they receive from family and friends who have stood by them over the years. Many have helped them financially as well as emotionally, but Ray continues to suffer from chronic ABS and Sierra has been diagnosed with PTSD. They are financially and emotionally bankrupt.

Ray's case points out how disruptive ABS can be on so many levels; legal, financial, emotional, relational, not to mention body-mind and gut-brain. So many of our patients suffered for years before even finding the diagnosis. Then they had to search for the medical and lifestyle treatments that worked for their unique individual being, but Ray hasn't found that combination yet.

He may need to try the "big guns" of the IV micafungin or even a fecal transplant before finding relief but he is not allowed to travel out of state. Meanwhile, Ray has long wait times for appointments and can only hope the VA will listen to doctors from other states. The fight goes on.

CHAPTER 15

A QUAGMIRE OF LEGAL ISSUES

You have the right to remain silent. Anything you say can and will be used against you in a court of law...

— *U.S. Miranda Warning*

There is no precedent for treating "drunk-without-drinking" as a medical disease in the legal arena. Several ABS patients have been acquitted of responsibility for their first DUI, others have resolved a charge by paying the fine or doing jail time or both. Still others are tangled in the legal system, embroiled in appeals. This is as unfair as blaming someone with a first-time seizure for an accident.

Laurie to Ray and Sierra: *Sorry, no good news from our end. We were called liars by initial DUI attorneys we interviewed. The one who took our case also took $10,000, then advised us to plea anyway because nobody had heard of the condition. This was 2011. A judge told me that since the ABC 20/20 show he is now aware of the illness but it's too late for us. Will keep you in our thoughts and hope for positive outcome.*

Ray and Sierra Lewis's story, as well as Laurie's, highlight the tragedy of our justice system when it fails to advocate for someone who is sick but doesn't yet know it. To have a judge acknowledge the disease and then tell you it's too late speaks to just how unresponsive the legal system really is. The impact for someone like Ray and Sierra is astronomical; virtually all aspects of their lives are damaged.

Sierra: *It's the legal persecution that I simply want to END. Going from healthy to disabled, losing your freedom to drive, needing someone to make sure you're alive, those are difficult enough. But to lose your entire life's work, your professional reputation, AND your home because the legal system decides you're a horrible criminal? That is what I cannot accept. Ever.*

In this case and many others, the scotoma in the medical and legal systems intersect by denying ABS exists even when presented with ample evidence. Prosecutors continue to cite the decades-old article out of Sweden I mentioned, and conveniently forget more recent cases and acquittals.

A woman in Hamburg, NY was arrested for DWI after having 4 drinks over nearly six hours. She submitted to a breathalyzer test which showed that her BrAC was nearly four times the legal limit (.30%). Due to the high BrAC reading they took her to the hospital. Following a physical examination wherein she appeared sober, the Emergency Department staff wanted to release her, but her husband requested they run a blood test. Five hours after her last drink her BAC registered .33%.

The woman's attorney, Joseph Marusak began sleuthing to try and explain this bizarre confluence of facts. At Marusak's direction the woman and her husband tested her BrAC every evening for nearly three weeks with a portable breathalyzer kit. She consistently registered a BrAC above .20 % despite her abstinence from alcoholic beverages.

Marusak then hired two nurses and a physician's assistant to conduct a twelve-hour controlled observation to ensure she was not drinking, during which time they drew three samples of her blood (9 AM, 6 PM and 8:30 PM). Pursuant to a court order the forensic lab used by the prosecution tested those samples. Bingo! Despite the woman's abstinence from alcohol all three samples registered a BAC well above the legal limit, with the last draw yielding a .36% BAC.

Marusak requested the woman to seek a diagnosis from Dr. Anup Kanodia, a nationally recognized expert from Columbus, Ohio, who concluded that she was afflicted with Auto-brewery Syndrome at the time of her arrest. In addition, Marusak retained a clinical pharmacologist who rendered an expert opinion that the woman's BAC level at the time of her arrest (based upon her consumption of four drinks over six hours) would have been within the range of .01 to .05 %, well below the legal limit.

Based on the above evidence, the court granted Marusak's motion to dismiss the criminal case in the interest of justice.[191]

Believe me, there is no way I would want someone with active ABS to drive. But a person should not be held responsible for a first-time driving violation due to a little-known, undiagnosed disease that can show up at a moment's notice with no warning.

Sierra: *Post-accident, Ray was passed from doctor to specialist to doctor again. After long and extensive testing and analysis, Ray was diagnosed with Auto Brewery Syndrome. At the time of this discovery, the State of Oregon was pursuing a case against Ray for the accident, amounting to Misdemeanor Driving Under the Influence (DUI) and Reckless Driving. Despite the medical evidence, they chose to challenge the findings.*

The resulting trial [January 2016] consisted of several days of proceedings. The first day involved testimony and evidence about ABS, and its relevance to this particular case. On that day, the Lane County court (Eugene, Oregon) acknowledged that Auto Brewery Syndrome was a legitimately diagnosed disease, and that they had the leading expert there that day for testimony.

They further acknowledged that Dr. Anup Kanodia (that leading expert, testifying after being sworn in) verified that Ray suffered from Auto Brewery Syndrome, from approximately October 2013, though no outright acute symptoms would have been observable at that time.

Despite this evidence, Judge Karrie McIntyre chose to invoke the shield of "Strict Liability." Strict Liability in DUI cases states that it doesn't matter how an individual becomes intoxicated; the bottom line is that they are. Without the Strict Liability law, anyone who is intoxicated could blame anyone else [like a bartender or the brewer] *and say it was someone else's fault.*

---

191   Marusak J. personal communication, February 21-26, 2019

Ray's case exemplifies that there are medical exceptions to the Strict Liability rule. And rare as they may be, they need to be examined. Undiagnosed diabetics and epileptics involved in vehicle accidents are exonerated immediately from all criminal proceedings once a medical diagnosis is discovered. These cases never make it to trial because the legal system recognizes that they are medical issues, not criminal actions.

What the short-sighted State of Oregon judge has failed to see is that this case would establish precedence regarding proof of Auto Brewery Syndrome diagnosis and that it bears distinction from DUI defendants grasping for a legal defense. The specific medical markers that identify Auto Brewery Syndrome cannot be faked. In addition to the inability to fabricate the disease and diagnosis, the exorbitant cost will deter anyone else from pursuing even the first phase of any legal proceedings that arise from a false claim of having Auto Brewery Syndrome.

This case clearly illustrates the legal quagmire that faces people who are arrested without knowing they have ABS. Ray and Sierra are still immersed in the appeals process.

ARRESTS AND DUIS

One of the most critical advocacy issues in dealing with ABS is the legal system. Many of our patients have received citations for DUI or DWI after only one drink or with nothing to drink. Some of our patients did not know they were suffering from gut fermentation until they received a ticket and knew they hadn't been drinking, and this trigger sent them on the hunt for a diagnosis.

While Barry Logan of Washington University and Alan Wayne Jones of Sweden judge the accounts of Japanese ABS cases as "reliable," they state, "this syndrome...has only ever been documented in Japanese people." [192] Really? Just one more reason I needed to write this book.

Then they conclude "after careful consideration and review of the current scientific literature...except in exceptional and well-defined

---

192   Logan B, Jones A. (2000) Endogenous ethanol: Auto-Brewery Syndrome" as a drunk-driving defence challenge. *Med Sci Law* 40(3):206-216

circumstances, it is not possible for a living person to generate sufficient amounts of ethanol in the body…to yield forensically significant concentrations in peripheral venous blood" (p.214). What? I call a foul! Can you spot the flaw in the logic?

Logan and Jones published their article, *Endogenous Ethanol: Auto-Brewery Syndrome as a Drunk-driving Defence Challenge* in 2000 and, sadly, many prosecutors still rely on the article in courts of law without looking at the numerous ABS cases published, and the plethora of science acquired in the last nineteen years.

I have no doubt that a few people have tried to get out of a DUI by falsely claiming a diagnosis of ABS but that doesn't mean it doesn't exist. Many of us believe ABS should be treated like a seizure disorder; if a person does not know he or she has ABS, the law should excuse them the first time the symptoms cause someone to inadvertently break a law. After that, the person should not drive or operate machinery until the condition is addressed or is brought under well-documented control for a time.

······

Sierra: (in response to a query regarding legalities of DUI and ABS): *Personally, Ray and I feel like once you know you have ABS, you shouldn't drive. At that point, you know you have a medical condition (even if the legal and medical systems don't acknowledge it). Ray stopped driving more than nine months before he officially lost his license because of the DUI case.*

We both realized that he was not medically safe to drive – just like a diabetic or an epileptic [uncontrolled] would be a danger. If Ray ever gets back to the point where he is asymptomatic for a very long period of time, we will reconsider it. Neither of us could live with ourselves if he got behind the wheel, flared, and someone died because of it.

Thankfully, other than Ray, very few of our patients have been involved in accidents or received DUIs. I haven't found any other articles linking ABS or even unexplained intoxication with DUIs or accidents. I have received several phone calls from attorneys wanting to know more about ABS as a possible defense, but I have only heard of a few success stories of acquittals in addition to the one Joe Marusak related to me.

Mostly, I get calls from people who got a DUI without drinking anything. That was their first clue that something was wrong with them. I refer them to the website to read the articles and list of doctors who can diagnose them. What a challenge for these folks.

Just like the medical establishment, the legal system needs to update their science and information and treat clients with an open mind. The ongoing challenge for advocates is to educate attorneys, prosecutors, and judges about ABS. But we must first update medical providers if we ever hope to inform the legal system.

CHAPTER 16

THE PUSH TOWARD BODY-MIND INTEGRATIVE MEDICINE

Not all things that count can be counted.

— *Larry Dossey, MD*

ABS bought me a front row seat at the long-standing competition between conventional medicine and integrative or holistic health. As a Board-Certified Holistic Nurse with a Ph.D., I know the body, mind, and spirit are inseparable and believe we should refer to the whole person and integrative medicine in any discussion of health or illness.

However, Rene Descartes did us a grave disservice in the 1640s when he concluded a dualistic distinction of the "immaterial mind" from the body.[193] Even though neurologists proved him wrong in short order, Descartes' legacy lives on in such a pervasive way that we still have scientists who only study the mind and others who study only the body.

Our medical culture continues to separate the body, the mind, and the spirit especially in healthcare. An example of the trichotomy is that people with mental illness are generally not treated in a medical hospital but are transferred to a mental hospital. And they may be transferred back if they have a physical ailment and discharged if they have a behavioral or spiritual crisis.

---

193   Descartes R. (2007) Meditations on First Philosophy in which are demonstrated the existence of God and the distinction between the human soul and body. Jonathan Bennett. https://philpapers.org/rec/BENLFS-2 Retrieved: 9-22-18

All maladies involve the body-mind-spirit sciences as we remember the chapter on the microbiome and the inter-relationships between the gut and the digestive, immune, endocrine, metabolic, and emotional systems. Even something as straightforward as a physical cut to your body involves the mind because pain signals are sent to and interpreted by your brain. Your mind may think about the cause of the laceration - *I was distracted.*

Your gut gets involved with immunity by protecting the cut from infection as it heals. And the gut as the second brain also relays and augments emotions and feelings such as frustration or guilt - *Why was I in such a hurry with that knife?* You may even struggle with a spiritual significance about the cut and the meaning of the pain - *I'm being punished.*

Some of these thoughts, feelings, and emotions may in turn affect your gut by the feedback loop of the sympathetic nervous system that initiates the fight or flight response also known as stress. The fight or flight response is a reflex of our sympathetic nervous system that activates in the face of danger.

A rush of adrenaline leads to increased heart rate and blood pressure to send extra blood to the muscles, increased breathing to send extra oxygen with the blood, and heightened awareness. Fight or flight diverts resources away from basic functions like digestion and immunity to enable us to respond to danger quickly; to run away from the tiger. It's what enables someone to lift a car off their baby in dire circumstances.

The stresses of a chronic illness or disease (or situation), may over time however, initiate a cascade of body-mind effects such as poor digestion, indigestion, constipation, shallow breathing, increased heart rate, poor quality sleep, nervousness, as well as increased irritability and muscle tension.[194]

---

194   Harvard Health Publishing (2018) Understanding the stress response. https://www.health. harvard.edu/staying-healthy/understanding-the-stress-response Retrieved: 10-12-18

M ind, body, and spirit are all involved in holistic medicine and treatments, but authors usually shorten the connection to "body-mind" with the all-important spiritual aspect getting the short shrift. Spirit connotes religion to many, but in a holistic approach spirit focuses on the important issues of life for all of us whether we are religious or not.

My favorite holistic nurse role models, Dr. Barbara Dossey and Dr. Lynn Keegan, discuss spirituality as including meaning that is considered sacred or holy, and interconnectedness with self, nature, others, and God or the transcendent. Nurturing the spiritual in us is shown to be essential to our well-being.[195] Our spiritual nature asks and finds answers to important questions like "Why am I here and what is my purpose?" "How am I connected to my higher power and others?" and "What gives me deep peace and joy?"

The term body-mind should not be confused with psychosomatic or somatoform disorders meaning physical ailments *caused* by mental factors. For example, chest pain may be caused by a belief that one has cardiac disease where no physical disease process is found. This is a true somatoform disorder. These terms often have a negative connotation such as "it's all in your head."

Body-mind or holistic medicine acknowledges the connection of all physical ailments with the mind and the spirit including functional disorders with no perceived cause. For example, some types of irritable bowel may be brought on by stress without another underlying disease process and this would be considered a functional disorder.

Because conventional medicine does not always have good answers for complex chronic conditions, many people turn to holistic, ancient, and traditional practices, like acupuncture, aromatherapy, and energy work. Fortunately, our language has evolved over the past few decades.

---

195   Dossey B, Keegan L. (2013) Holistic Nursing: A Handbook for Practice. Burlington, MA: Jones & Bartlett Learning

What was once called "quackery" by the modern medical doctors then became "unproven". Those terms gave way to terms like "questionable practices," and finally in the late twentieth century, traditional practices such as home remedies, homeopathy, massage, and plant medicine, finally earned the moniker "alternative medicine."

The research of the last twenty years on holistic modalities shows they are often effective as "complementary medicine;" that is, used along with conventional medicine. Even Congress funded the National Center for Complementary and Alternative Therapy (NCCAM) at the National Institutes of Health for the study of holistic practices; then later changed the name to the National Center for Complementary and Integrative Health (NCCIH).[196] Though it seems NCCIH still cannot quite settle on its name; is it complementary or integrative?

The hope is that someday our Western healthcare culture will be able to practice "integrative medicine and wellness" by embracing conventional medicine and holistic activities in the same breath and practice.

But for now, the friction between modern medical practice and holistic or integrative medicine remains quite charged. Practitioners are not the only ones who are conflicted about the other end of their trained spectrum; patients often bounce back and forth between conventional and holistic treatments. Let's peek behind the curtain of these two positions, conventional medicine and holistic practices, to better understand how to integrate them in an effective way.

A GLIMPSE AT THE HISTORY
OF CONVENTIONAL MEDICINE

Modern conventional medicine has evolved greatly in the past 100 years but now consists largely of diagnosis and treatment with medications, surgery, and radiation. If we include mental illness as part of this category,

---

196   National Center for Complementary and Integrative Health. https://nccih.nih.gov/about

we can add psychotherapy and electroconvulsive therapy (ECT) to the list of treatments.

Prior to the Civil War, anyone in the United States could practice medicine. There were many private medical schools throughout the country and a high ratio of what were called "doctors" to people – up to 175 doctors per 100,000 people. The current system of conventional medicine developed in the West during the late nineteenth century as medical schools became more grounded in science. In 1893, Johns Hopkins Medical School was founded and became the standard for science-based medicine.

People don't realize it was just 100 years ago that The Federation of Medical Boards started issuing and requiring a license to practice medicine. Licenses are required ostensibly to protect the public with minimum standards of practice for physicians. Practice?

The dual meaning of the word "practice" in the Merriam-Webster Dictionary is interesting because while I believe doctors "pursue their profession" they should also "perform or work at repeatedly, to improve performance." How many physicians really continue to practice in order to improve? Often, continuing education consists of a lecture followed by an afternoon of skiing (yes, I'm jealous of the skiing write-off).

Abraham Flexner, an educator, reported in 1910,[197] on the state of American medical education which helped intensify the reform of medical schools towards a Johns Hopkins-model. The report remonstrated the deficient education offered in many medical schools and within a decade 30 percent of American medical schools had closed.

This is when state medical boards began popping up to develop stringent regulations to standardize curricula, testing, and licensure. Of course, this process required money to attend an approved school and pay for a licensure exam, and thus the boards held great power over the practice of medicine.

---

197   Flexner A. (1910) Medical education in America: Rethinking the training of American doctors. *The Atlantic.* https://www.theatlantic.com/magazine/archive/1910/06/medical-education-in-america/306088/

Suddenly medicine became a business opportunity and investors began to bankroll regulatory agencies, research institutes, and pharmaceuticals. Now money infiltrates every aspect of medicine from research and development to testing and patents. We spend twice as much on healthcare in the United States than 10 other high-income countries.

Most of the difference comes from higher physician payments and higher cost of medicine. For example, the average salary for a general practice physician in the 10 other countries was between $86,607 and $154,126. In the US, the average physician salary was $218,173. Per capita spending for prescription drugs in other nations ranged from $466 to $939 but in the U.S., per capita spending was $1,443.[198]

Those extraordinary profits are going into the pockets of physicians and pharmaceutical executives as well as investors. Today, this influence of money and regulation (read power) continue to drive a wedge between medicine and science in the United States.

······

We don't have to look very far to find instances where money determines medical practice instead of science. In her 2018 book *Natural Causes*,[199] Barbara Ehrenreich recounts the story of being diagnosed with a disease that had no science behind it. She was cajoled into having a bone density scan after being told of the possibility of breaking a hip. Her test resulted in a diagnosis of 'osteopenia' and her doctor prescribed medication.

It turns out that osteopenia is a normal feature of aging and Ehrenreich discovered that bone density testing has been "heavily promoted and even subsidized by the drug's manufacturer" (p.4). It was a drug looking for a disease. Despite there being no further studies planned to prove the efficacy of

198   The Guardian. (2018). Sky-high prices of everything make US healthcare the world's most expensive. https://www.theguardian.com/us-news/2018/mar/13/us-healthcare-costs-causes-drug-prices-salaries Retrieved 10-15-18

199   Ehrenreich B, (2018) *Natural Causes: An epidemic of wellness, the certainty of dying, and killing ourselves to live longer.* New York:12

these drugs for this normal condition, doctors continue to prescribe the drug in record numbers. So much for science competing with profit.

And here's an example of the lack of science in medicine. If you've ever had general anesthesia, you may remember it took a few days to rebound from the groggy feeling in your brain. That's because tests on inhaled anesthetics show them to be toxic to the cells that control memory and learning, and even present Alzheimer's-like changes in mice.

General Anesthesia (GA) puts one into a reversible coma; we have no clear idea of the long-term effects of GA because it has *rarely been studied*. One 2012 study did show that children anesthetized for surgery before the age of three are twice as likely to develop learning disabilities by age ten. Nevertheless, doctors have used anesthesia for over 200 years without understanding how it works.

One author says, "...despite all the progress that has been made, we still lack a clear and comprehensive insight into the specific neurophysiological mechanisms of general anesthesia, from the molecular level to the global brain propagation."[200] And only in the last two decades have we come to realize that GA works by binding onto central nervous system cell receptors.[201] Remember the concept of prematurity? Here it is, big time!

No doubt, everyone who has ever had surgery is glad anesthesia is available, but my point is that doctors don't wait around for science to prove how something works, or even *that* it works. They dive right in and use what they believe to be good and in the best interest of patients. Often that belief backfires.

Let's take a short dive into mivacurium, commonly known as Versed, a neuromuscular-blocking drug (meaning paralytic) developed in the early 1980s. Paralytics are used in conjunction with GA to induce a coma with

200   Uhrug L, Dhaene S, Jarraya B. (2014) Cerebral mechanisms of general anesthesia. ISSN: 1769-6623. Feb; 33 (2):72-82 Elsevier; PMID: 24368069

201   Borelli L. (2015) https://www.medicaldaily.com/general-anesthesia-8-interesting-facts-about-procedure-puts-you-sleep-356872 Retrieved: 10-15-18

memory loss during short procedures such as colonoscopies, cardiac catheterizations, and removal of cataracts.

Versed has several untoward side effects including histamine release with resultant bronchospasm and hypotension in addition to well documented *residual paralysis!* [emphasis mine].[202] Supposedly due to supply-related manufacturing issues, the drug disappeared from the U.S. market in 2006.

A quick Medline search revealed over 10,000 articles on Versed and most of them appeared to be reports and research on negative side effects. Yet the manufacturer, AbbVie, Inc. of GlaxoSmithKline, reintroduced Versed in 2016. Why is the science being ignored? Do you think profit by the drug company might be a factor? Do you think those who use Versed even know all this?

Where is the science on anesthesia in general? It's basically medical science that has been experimenting on all of us for two centuries. We've gone from alcohol and ether to ketamine, midazolam and propofol to very sophisticated designer drugs that most of us cannot even pronounce. But after the rats (maybe), the patients become the research subjects, without informed consent, so doctors can compare drugs to each other and stop using the old ones. What do you think is driving this process?

••••••

Remember drugs like Vioxx for the pain of Rheumatoid Arthritis and Zelnorm for IBD with constipation that caused an increased risk of heart attack? Other drugs like Accutane for acne carried an increased risk of irritable bowel disease (IBD), and Darvon and Darvocet for acute pain were linked to cardiac toxicity. Before that, there was the horrific DES (diethylstilbestrol) which prevented miscarriage but caused birth defects.[203] All these medicines were recalled.

---

202   Soto R., et al. (2017) Mivacurium: Return of a drug seeking an indication? *ASA Monitor.* 81:30-31 http://anesthesiaexperts.com/uncategorized/mivacurium-return-drug-seeking-indication/ Retrieved: 10-15-18

203   Prescription Drugs. https://prescriptiondrugs.procon.org/view.resource. php?resourceID=005528 Retrieved 10-15-18

Too often drugs are produced, distributed, and marketed before being thoroughly tested. The motive is clearly profit! The lack of ethical testing for drugs is a huge indictment of the medical-industrial complex that most of us ignore.

The FDA pulled the previously mentioned medications and many others from the market, but only after they are involved in or have settled class action lawsuits. Even when the FDA removes a drug from the market and fines the manufacturer, it's a slap on the wrist compared with the windfall lucre already direct deposited in CEO and shareholders' pockets.

White Coat, Black Hat: Adventures on the Dark Side of Medicine by Carl Elliott is a fascinating read detailing a few complicit doctors who aid the pharmaceutical industry with shoddy drug testing.[204] Pharmaceutical companies spend billions of dollars to ensure that doctors know about their drugs and this is another way that money and influence pressure medical decision-making.

The multi-billion-dollar pharmaceutical industry disregards public health for profit with alarming regularity and convinces doctors to keep prescribing their drugs. There is also a revolving door between Big Pharma and the FDA so that decision-makers can loosen regulations on testing methods. This whole chain breeds a culture of apathy toward the very real health consequences for the public, but the money keeps rolling in.

••••••

The massive barge of medical education is also slow to change course, even in the face of significant evidence that contradicts standard practices. For example, when I went to nursing school, doctors and nurses were using hydrogen peroxide (H_2O_2) to clean wounds as a routine practice and I venture to say that most families followed the practice at home.

In the 1980s we learned from new research to use soap and water on a wound and skip the H_2O_2. While many of us spread the word, my latest

---

204   Elliott C. (2011) White Coat Black Hat: Adventures on the dark side of medicine. Boston: Beacon Press

library search revealed dozens of articles authored as recently as 2011 recommending the use of hydrogen peroxide in wound care. The authors apparently did not read the scientific journals and I still run across doctors who use and recommend hydrogen peroxide for wounds and scrapes!

If it takes this long to change the practice of simple wound care, think how long it will take to accept holistic medicine, which has often been effectively healing people for thousands of years.

HOLISTIC PRACTICES

I would be hard-pressed to come up with an accurate list of treatments that are considered alternative to our conventional medical treatments. Typically, holistic or alternative medicine is anything aside from conventional surgery, medication, and radiation.

I believe most people would agree that acupuncture, Reiki, and Ayurveda are still considered alternative. However, only two decades ago, nutrition, chiropractic, and probiotics were considered alternative by many in medicine. Now doctors routinely prescribe chiropractic care and discuss and recommend special diets and supplements such as probiotics for many ailments.

The term "alternative" is also used as a rubber stamp to describe anything not paid for by health insurance. Or is it code to keep insurance from covering the modality? Unfortunately, many effective modalities such as probiotics, chiropractic, and massage, are not covered or are only partially covered by insurance, even when recommended by a physician.

According to Reuters Health, "the U.S. spends about twice what other high-income nations do on health care but has the lowest life expectancy and the highest infant mortality rates."[205] In addition, conventional medicine does not have good answers for chronic issues so it's no wonder we turn to holistic modalities.

---

205   Rappaport L. (2018) U.S. health spending twice other countries with worse results. Reuters: https://www.reuters.com/article/us-health-spending/u-s-health-spending-twice-other-countries-with-worse-results-idUSKCN1GP2YN Retrieved: 11-25-18

Americans spent a whopping $30.2 billion out-of-pocket on holistic health approaches (or 9.2% of all out-of-pocket health expenses), according to a nationwide survey by the National Center for Complementary and Integrative Health in 2012.[206] The survey collected information on the use of many complementary health approaches, including dietary supplements, chiropractic or osteopathic manipulation, yoga, massage, and meditation.

Acupuncture is a good example of the difficulty of gaining acceptance by conventional medicine. Acupuncture is used in China for pain management and anesthesia and has been for centuries. A number of scientific studies show the effectiveness, and it boasts many avid proponents.

Stephen Birch and colleagues from the Foundation for the Study of East Asian Medicine in Amsterdam, Netherlands conducted meta-analyses of research articles on acupuncture. They concluded that:

> Acupuncture appears to be effective for postoperative dental pain, postoperative nausea and vomiting, and chemotherapy-related nausea and vomiting. For migraine, low-back pain, and temporomandibular disorders the results are considered positive by some and difficult to interpret by others. For a number of conditions such as fibromyalgia, osteoarthritis of the knee, and tennis elbow the evidence is considered promising, but more and better-quality research is needed. For conditions such as chronic pain, neck pain, asthma, and drug addiction the evidence is considered inconclusive and difficult to interpret. For smoking cessation, tinnitus, and weight loss the evidence is usually regarded as negative.[207]

More recently, researchers in China used functional Magnetic Resonance Imaging (fMRI) to reveal the neural mechanisms of acupuncture.

---

206   NCCIM (2016) Americans spent $30.2 billion Out of Pocket on Complementary Health Approaches. https://nccih.nih.gov/news/press/cost-spending-06222016 Retrieved: 11-26-18

207   Birch S, Hesselink J, Jonkman F, et al. (2004) Clinical research on acupuncture part 1: What have reviews of the efficacy of acupuncture told us so far? *Journal of Alternative and Complementary Medicine* 10(3):468-480

They showed that Acupuncture not only affects brain activity, but also modulates the connectivity of the brain. Acupuncture at disease-related acupoints influences disease-related brain regions and Acupuncture regulates the brain network that overlaps with pain-related areas.[208]

However, two doctors conclude in an editorial that acupuncture is "theatrical placebo" and "...should, ideally, be tested separately for effectiveness for each individual condition for which it has been proposed."[209] Really? I am not saying that acupuncture is conclusively more effective than anesthesia or medications, only that there is a double standard when medicine holds holistic therapies to incredibly high testing standards that it's not applying to its own accepted practices.

······

If we are going to acknowledge just how little research there is for conventional medicine to back its practices, we must also admit that holistic practices have even less. All human study has research challenges, but holistic medicine is fraught with additional measurement difficulties alluded to in the opening quote "Not all things that count can be counted."

Excellent credible clinicians and scientists are researching holistic modalities, but "the devil is in the details." Holistic practices are generally not regulated, and training can vary widely. Physicians, chiropractors, nurses, massage therapists, and others are regulated by licensure, but only six states require acupuncturists to have a license. Energy workers and Ayurveda practitioners have no regulation at all. How do we know that what one person receives in a Reiki session is even close to what another receives?

Measurement is the largest barrier to researching holistic methods. For example, medicines are regulated by the U.S. Food and Drug Administration (FDA), but herbs and supplements do not have an equivalent regulatory

---

208   He T, Zhu W, Du S, et al. (2015) Neural mechanisms of acupuncture as revealed by fMRI studies. *Autonomic Neuroscience* 190:1-9 https://doi.org/10.1016/j.autneu.2015.03.006

209   Colquhoun D, Novella S. (2013) Acupuncture is theatrical placebo. *International Anesthesia Research Society* 116(6):1360-1363 DOI: 10.1213/ANE.0b013e31828f2d5e

body. We don't always know what's really in a bottle of "bone health" even when we read the ingredients – where is the quality control?

There's no standardization of herbal medicines and other supplements. If you've ever looked at probiotics, for example, you find dozens of brands with scores of species and millions or billions of microbes. And why the secretive "proprietary blends?"

If one brand with five species of three billion microbes each is tested in a double-blind study, that doesn't mean all brands of probiotics will work the same way. After exploring the microbiome, you understand why. And think of the money it would take to research even a fraction of all the supplements on the market.

Standardizing and quantifying treatments like acupuncture, aromatherapy, and energy work are even more difficult than measuring herbs and supplements. There are challenges to measurement not just with interventions but also with outcomes. How do we measure energy or hope as an outcome? Why do we continue to discount the placebo effect that many people feel better even if a medicine has no active ingredient? Belief is powerful in healing!

Another difficulty is that most health outcomes are subjective. Researchers measure pain and anxiety with a 10-point scale but even that is subjective. We know that self-report isn't always accurate, but how else can we get rigorous information on human behavior over time?

Trying to measure outcomes with subjective qualities like relaxation or spiritual well-being is even harder. These types of healing modalities also straddle physical medicine and psychology – body-mind – so how do we measure both?

Richard Nahin and Stephen Straus, directors at NCCIH, acknowledge the research difficulties as well as the potential of research into therapies already widely in use by consumers.[210] One challenge is the complex, individualized treatments being used. Rarely do practitioners recommend, or

---

210   Nahin R, Straus S. (2001) Research into complementary and alternative medicine: problems and potential. *BMJ* 322(7279):161-164 https://www.ncbi.nlm.nih.gov/pmc/articles/PMC1119420/

patients choose, one therapy at a time, but they often mix herbs, supplements, massage, and other modalities.

Research design is a challenge anytime we study human health that we know is largely influenced by behavior and lifestyle choices. All human research involves these last two difficulties. The first is identifying appropriate placebo interventions. A placebo for a medication is a lot easier to find than something to mimic, say, a massage or a chiropractic adjustment.

The second challenge is recruiting, randomizing, and retaining patients. Finding subjects with the factor being studied who are willing to participate is a huge issue. There are many reasons people don't choose to participate in research, including time, incentive, and fear to name a few. Researchers struggle with the idea that people who participate may differ in some basic way from those who choose not to participate.

Researchers must have large numbers of subjects for sound research design in randomizing subjects, but this increases the cost of a study. And lastly, subjects may drop out of the research for a myriad of reasons so retaining them is difficult.

And remember, there is very little incentive for scientists to study something that is already amassing great wealth for the businesses promoting unregulated supplements, therapies, and superfoods. Money drives research and even the researchers need to get paid.

In summary, conventional medicine and holistic modalities each have much to offer patients and consumers. We must continue to integrate the two schools of thought to improve treatments for difficult and obscure syndromes as well as promoting wellness. We need watchdog groups to ensure science and not money motivates conventional and holistic practices, as well as research.

CHAPTER 17

TRIAL AND ERROR: TREATING ABS

Medical science has proven time and again that when the resources are provided, great progress in the treatment, cure, and prevention of disease can occur.

— *Michael J. Fox*

In this chapter I will discuss the major elements of treatment for ABS. I've also put together a bulleted list in Appendix B of the diagnosis and treatment as a handy reference.

WASHOUT

The immediate concern for someone with ABS is safety. Caregivers must try to prevent injury during a flare. If still functioning, the patient may just need to be watched and encouraged to rest and sleep if possible. Alcohol causes dehydration and lowers blood sugar and a caregiver may need to encourage the patient to replace fluids and eat complex carbohydrates - leafy greens, remember? - or protein and fat to slowly raise blood sugar.

Someone with a BAC of 0.3% or higher is essentially poisoned and in danger of death. Alcohol is a central nervous system depressant and can cause respiratory arrest. A patient at this level of intoxication may be comatose and should be placed in a side-lying position to prevent choking in the event of vomiting. You should seek medical attention.

In a hospital or clinic, the provders will prescribe IV fluids for dehydration. The fluids will likely contain electrolytes and vitamins to replace those lost during intoxication, poisoning, and detox. The patient's cardiac, respiratory, and neurological vital signs will also be closely monitored until the flare subsides.

Just as important is support during the period immediately after the flare we call "washout." The washout is similar to a hangover for some ABS patients but can be quantitatively and qualitatively different. Most people can recover from a night of heavy drinking in about 24 hours. But for a person with ABS, the washout can linger for days. Our patients describe:

- Facial flushing, headaches, nausea, vomiting, and a rapid heart rate (like a hangover)

- Days of detox symptoms: shaking, chills, fever

- Lethargy; extreme tiredness; lack of energy; sleepy but unable to sleep

- Bad breath; bad taste in the mouth

- Joint pain and muscle aches

- Extremely irritable bowel issues including diarrhea, distention, belching, and flatulence

- Dehydration

- Blood pressure and pulse fluctuations; irregular pulse

- Lack of appetite

- Disrupted sleep

- Depression

People with ABS may experience any or all these symptoms after any flare. That must be horrible for someone experiencing flares every few days. Caregivers also must wade through this process, not only supporting the patient physically and emotionally, but often picking up the tasks and activities the patient is too sick to handle.

TREATMENT

The treatment for ABS ranges across the entire spectrum from conventional medications to lifestyle management to holistic treatments. Some ABS patients respond to integrative combinations of these three options including:

- Antifungals such as fluconazole, nystatin, or IV micafungin
- Low carbohydrate diet such as FODMAP, anti-candida diet, South Beach, or Keto
- Abstinence from alcohol in all forms
- Probiotic foods and supplements
- Supplements that support gut health such as grapefruit seed extract
- Stress reduction
- Environmental redesign to avoid toxins and other known triggers

Provider-patient collaboration is an essential part of treatment since individuals respond differently to various treatments. Donato was fortunate to have a team of providers including an infectious disease doctor who could prescribe medications, an endocrinologist who helped manage his diabetes in light of his ABS, a nutritionist who recommended dietary changes, and other integrative care providers. You should request referrals and information-sharing so that care planning is centered around the patient.

Remarkably, many patients use the word "cured," although perhaps with an inhale of the breath because many know through experience that relapse is a real threat looming in a small percentage of sufferers. I have talked to patients who resolved their symptoms with diet, abstinence from alcohol, and lifestyle changes alone. They affirm these changes have eliminated their ABS symptoms knowing they must maintain the new lifestyle.

Some patients follow the path of conventional western medicine with its prescriptions for anti-fungal medications and a low carbohydrate diet and probiotics and have no more symptoms. Other patients took numerous courses of medications and finally got relief when they made more comprehensive diet and lifestyle changes. Sadly, a few patients have tried every avenue open to them for treatment without relief.

It appears that ABS is one of those conditions, much like Lyme disease or Hepatitis B, which can be "acute" and ultimately resolved, or can become "chronic" with lifelong disability. Some in the chronic group can manage their symptoms with only a few flares per year while others, like Nick and Ray, continue to suffer greatly with frequent flares.

Our band of citizen scientists advocate in an ongoing battle to find effective treatments. We ask doctors, physician assistants, nurse practitioners, nurses, nutritionists, dentists, researchers, and anyone else in the health field who will listen to us, to help us generate more answers in the GI and microbiome treatment arena.

Our patients are the real-life laboratory and help one another discover and try various mainstream and holistic therapies. Collectively, we are sharing and finding connections and various regimens that work for many ABS sufferers; the most prominent and successful approaches are described here.

MEDICATIONS

The published articles on ABS prior to 1990 describe the effective use of antibiotic and antifungal medications. Kaji et al. detailed 39 case reports from Japan in the literature and the medical treatment with oral gentian violet, Trichomycin, and nystatinum.[211]

The authors claim that "most cases [are] easily cured by the administration of antifungal agents such as Trichomycin, Amphotericin B, or mycostatin." They go on to say that some cases resolve spontaneously but that ten of

---

211   Kaji H, Asunuma Y, Yahara O, et al. (1984) Intragastrointestinal Gut Fermentation Syndrome: Report of Two Cases and Review of Literature. *J Foren Sci Soc* 24(5):461-471

the 39 cases required surgical removal of the site of fermentation. I assume they mean they removed part of the small or large intestines, but the articles do not give details of the surgeries.

The big guns against intestinal yeast today are still the azole class of antifungal medications such as oral or IV fluconazole (Diflucan) and voriconazole (Vfend), and the polyene class of oral nystatin (Nystop, Nyata). You may be familiar with nystatin because it also comes in a tube for topical treatment of fungal skin infections.

The course of treatment with these two classes of medications are typically higher and longer for ABS treatment than those used for other types of fungal infections. Amphotericin B is also in the polyene class but is rarely used except in life-threatening infections due to the serious side effects. Micafungin sodium is a semi-synthetic echinocandin (a new class of anti-fungal) and was used in the Staten Island case.

Dr. McCarthy prescribed Joe a course of oral fluconazole 100mg a day for three weeks followed by nystatin 500,000 IU three times a day for three weeks. The medication regimen along with diet, probiotics and lifestyle changes, worked for him and other patients whose doctors have followed it.

Stacey followed the same medication and diet regimen with relief after Larry insisted the doctors read the case study and prescribe the meds. But Donato did not respond to any of the azoles or nystatin and required a very long course of IV micafungin sodium (Mycamine).

Since the Kaji article, I have not seen a published article that used Amphotericin B but maybe some doctors are prescribing it for ABS and have not published their cases.

We know that some yeasts, like Donato's are resistant to common anti-fungals. If the patient is not responding to medication, it is important for the medical providers to take samples from the gut and obtain laboratory DNA confirmation of the type of yeast. They should also perform sensitivity studies to determine which antifungal will be most effective. Donato's doctors ended up using micafungin.

Physicians, nurses and pharmacists are always aware of a potential for an allergic reaction and if a patient has an allergic reaction the doctor will have to prescribe another medication. All medications have some unfavorable side effects that vary from person to person. The table below lists the untoward side effects for the three major antifungal classes used for ABS.

Polyenes (i.e. nystatin):	Azoles (i.e. fluconazole):	Echinocandins (i.e. micafungin):
• Dry mouth • Rash • Upset stomach • Nausea • Vomiting • Diarrhea	• Too numerous to list but the most common are: • Headache • Upset stomach • Hair loss • Changes in renal and hepatic function	• Nausea & vomiting • Stomach pain • Indigestion • Diarrhea • Constipation • Headache • Insomnia • Body Flushing (blood rushing to the skin)

If you are a provider reading this, we sometimes need you to take treatment beyond the published studies. Design a plan of treatment specific to each patient. Call the team in Staten Island to learn how they treated Donato. Please, think outside the box and try combinations of medications and integrate holistic recommendations.

DIET AND DIET THERAPY

Nearly every treatment plan, with or without medication includes some form of a low carbohydrate diet. Some people choose a low glycemic index diet, while others use a more prescriptive diet such as South Beach, Whole 30, FODMAP, the Candida Diet, or Ketogenic Diet using clean meats without hormones, antibiotics, and chemical preservatives.

Sugars and carbohydrates should be severely restricted while the patient is on medication and even a few weeks beyond, but most patients are able to add a few carbohydrates back into their diet once symptoms resolve. Many of our patients adopt a low glycemic diet for life with only periodic treats of a dessert or a high glycemic pleasure like potatoes, rice, or bread.

Remember that I encourage patients to keep a journal of activities, food, and BAC, and try to determine which foods trigger flares? This is when the logbook becomes invaluable – during treatment. A pattern will emerge to show you what foods trigger a flare, so you know what to eliminate.

The journal or logbook can offer helpful clues, but the best way to really know what foods to eat is to go on an elimination diet and then slowly add back foods to see if there is a reaction or flare. Much like detecting food sensitivities or allergies, one would eliminate all obvious offending foods.

For ABS patients, you usually start by eating organic clean meat and organic green leafy vegetables. After a one to three-week cleansing period, you would start adding in one food at a time to see if you flare. Even if you experience bloating or gas without a flare, that may indicate a food sensitivity and you may want to eliminate that food for the time being.

Some patients have discovered they cannot eat dairy, but others can; still others can only eat fermented dairy such as yogurt and kefir. Some patients have realized they cannot eat sugars or artificial sweeteners of any kind, while others can ingest certain types of sugar and not others.

One patient I worked with flared with high fructose corn syrup but not regular sugar. Others can eat honey but not refined sugar. Some patients find they can eat very little variety of food at all and may, in fact, have food intolerances along with ABS.

Foods such as coffee, cheese, and peanuts can harbor mold; these are also triggers for many patients. Most patients avoid their personal triggers even after a cure, just because they feel better.

Michelle and Donato learned which foods he could and could not eat through the trial and learning curve of an elimination diet:

- *Fatty diets feed the yeast - only lean protein - fish is the best and easiest to digest*

- *Bread, pasta, rice, potatoes and any desserts/sugar can cause extreme rise in his BAC*

- *Animal protein brings the alcohol level down and keeps it down*

- *Only eat low glycemic veggies with animal protein. Veggies that he can eat are green; the only exceptions - no peas, but yes for cauliflower*

- *Cheese is good. Low carb yogurt is good*

Here is an example of the elimination diet from Julia. She is a registered nutritionist and had difficulty recommending a diet for her husband because each book she read had different recommendations for re-balancing yeast: *B. is basically eating meat and non-starchy vegetables. We did not eliminate coffee, tea, or vinegar (because B. loves mustard and hot sauce). However, given that the episodes have not let up, we are changing approaches.*

We are going to follow The Candida Cure diet faithfully, including eliminating coffee, tea, and vinegar. This diet is more liberal on some things (allows small amounts of beans and sweet potatoes and winter squash and some gluten-free grain substitutes such as quinoa, for example), so after months of meat and veggies, having some of these again will be quite welcome in our house.

And another perspective from Sierra: *It's taken years to stock our pantry with things that I can grab quickly and make healthy meals that Ray can enjoy. Homemade pressure-canned turkey stock, garden fresh kale and onions, and a brand of chicken apple sausage that Ray can eat safely in moderation. Changing my way of thinking about food combos has taken awhile, but when it works it is highly satisfying.*

A NOTE ABOUT ALCOHOL

I tell every ABS patient and family member I work with the unvarnished truth: someone who has ABS or is cured of ABS should not drink alcohol again – EVER. I hate to tell people the bad news because it's such an avenue of pleasure for so many people, but during ABS treatment, the patient who drinks is counteracting the antifungals. And if you had ABS but you are asymptomatic, you are just asking for trouble.

The main reason that I strongly suggest avoiding alcohol is that the diet and drugs do not eliminate fermenting yeast from our guts during treatment. Treatment and management only return these yeasts to a commensal balance. Based on the science, we don't want to eliminate yeast because of the beneficial functions they perform. But somehow, the fermenting yeast that remain in the gut seem to be stimulated by ethanol and can easily grow out of control once again.

As long as we can't explain this response, and so many patients experience the extremely high BACs with drinking only one or two drinks, it is my professional opinion that drinking is poking the anthill. Patients who think they can drink moderately again often find themselves in the throes of a relapse. It's simply not worth the risk.

PREBIOTICS, PROBIOTICS
AND OTHER HOLISTIC TREATMENTS

Now that you've read about the microbiome and disturbances in the microbiome, it is evident why there is such a fervor over live beneficial cultures. And you can see why it is difficult to select effective ones during ABS treatment. You can also understand why there is an explosion of unregulated probiotic sales in the form of pills and fermented superfoods.

But is it sauerkraut and yogurt that's going to save us, or is it powders and capsules? As Karen said, *you could go mad trying every potential cure out there.*

Prebiotics are foods such as greens, onions, garlic, bananas and other high fiber foods that feed the microorganisms in our guts to promote healthy balance. They are like fertilizer for the soil in our garden. Our ABS support populace of patients and caregivers also report adding fermented foods to their diets for the prebiotic effect.

Probiotics are foods such as yogurt, kefir and sauerkraut or supplements in pill or powder form that contain *live* microorganisms intended to maintain or improve the microbiome. They are like adding more good seeds to our garden. Many of our treating physicians and nutritionists have recommended probiotics as part of the treatment regimen.

Many patients choose their own probiotics even if not recommended by their doctor or nutritionist. Isn't it ironic that fermented foods can help halt over-fermentation in the gut? Obviously, the jury is still out as to which probiotics are most effective for ABS, but many of our patients and their healthcare providers are willing to try anything to help reverse this devastating syndrome.

······

Numerous studies examine the effectiveness of probiotics on liver disease, autism spectrum disorder, allergic disorders, and especially GI disorders such as SIBO, IBS and IBD. However, researchers have not yet determined which specific probiotics are best, or how to quantify dosages. According to the National Institutes of Health, "The U.S. Food and Drug Administration (FDA) has not approved any probiotic for treating or preventing any disease."

Their website states:

Because many research studies on probiotics haven't looked closely at safety, there isn't enough information right now to answer some safety questions. Most of our knowledge about safety comes from studies of *Lactobacillus* and *Bifidobacterium*; less is known about other probiotics. Information on the long-term safety of probiotics is limited, and safety may differ from one type of probiotic to another. For example, even though a National Center for Complementary and Integrative Health (NCCIH)-funded study showed that a particular kind of *Lactobacillus* appears safe in healthy adults age 65 and older, this does not mean that all probiotics would necessarily be safe for people in this age group.[212]

A few studies are showing promising results, however. A systematic review evaluated fifteen randomized, double-blind studies that examined the power of probiotics in the treatment of lactose intolerance (LI) and showed varying degrees of efficacy but an overall positive effect of the use of probiotics in LI.[213]

Dr. Annina Zihler and three other food scientists in Zurich, Switzerland showed that probiotics provide protective effects against *Salmonella* infectivity in an in vitro gut fermentation model and hold promise for developing novel antimicrobials.[214]

According to University of Calgary scientists Vrinda Nair and Amuchou Soraisham, the common microorganisms used in probiotics include a) Bacteria: *Lactobacillus rhamnosus, L. acidophilus, L. caseii, L. plantaru, L. lactis,* etc.; *Bifidobacter bifidum, B. brefis, B. infantis,* etc.; *Steptococcus thermophiles*; and b) Yeast: *Saccharomyces boulardii.*[215] They reviewed several articles that demonstrate preventive effects in preterm infants. Be careful though, because *S. boulardii* can become invasive and infect the bloodstream under certain conditions. You should thoroughly research your products and consult with a nutritionist if you have concerns.

······

M any of our citizen scientists search probiotics online and share recommendations with each other. The anecdotal evidence for reversing ABS with only diet and probiotics or adding probiotics and other supplements to

---

212   National Center for Complementary and Integrative Health https://nccih.nih.gov/health/probiotics/introduction.htm Retrieved on 8-23-18

213   Oak S, Jha R. (2018) The effects of probiotics in lactose intolerance: A systematic review. *Crit Rev in Food Sci & Nutr.* https://doi.org/10.1080/10408398.2018.1425977

214   Zihler A, Gagnon M, Chassard C, Lacroix C. (2011) Protective effect of probiotics on Salmonella infectivity assessed with combined in vitro gut fermentation-cellular models. *BMC Micro* 11:264 https://doi.org/10.1186/1471-2180-11-264

215   Nair V, Soraisham A. (2013) Probiotics and Prebiotics: Role in prevention of nosocomial sepsis in preterm infants. *Intl J Pedi* http://dx.doi.org/10.1155/2013/874726

a medication regimen is promising so far. Here are a couple of our caregivers' thoughts:

Christina: *Great news we think! After six weeks of Diflucan and nystatin and tons of probiotics, S. was instructed by our Dr. to resume a normal diet. He's blown zeros this week. We are so happy for each day he's a zero and hoping it will last.*

Winter: *In addition to the antifungal medication and the candida cleanse, we added a multitude of probiotics and supplements: turmeric, curcumin, selenium, and NAC* [N-acetyl cysteine] *(NAC helped my husband's mental state, depression, and confusion).*

I would highly recommend adding Chelated Molybdenum to your diet because it helps adhere to the toxins that build up but cannot be excreted; this was important for us, if we thought he was about to have an episode we would double up on the dose. We added a probiotic as well.

INTEGRATED TREATMENT FOR ABS

Many of our ABS patients use Conventional medicine as well as Holistic modalities and are often able to integrate the two quite seamlessly. Here is an example from a caregiver: *He hasn't blown a positive yet all week! Is my husband cured?! Blood tests are all normal. We get breath test results on the 14th. We have done the following: Drugs, Chitin candida cleanse, Bone broth, strict GAPS and Candida diet for 4 months.*

In addition to probiotics, many of our patients tried enzymes and other supplements with varying degrees of success. Several of our ABS patients used grapefruit seed extract and other supplements with some success. I could find only one study of grapefruit seed extract that showed promise in a small sample of patients with intestinal dysbiosis.[216]

Gordon: *Grapefruit seed extract (GSE), has an antifungal nature and is available as an OTC supplement. As for GSE singularly, I cannot say that it has been my "cure," but I have to credit it with helping as I am currently not on any specific diet or drug protocol, so there is that.*

---

216   Ionescu F, Kiehl R, Wichmann-Kunz F, et al. (1990) Oral citrus seed extract in atopic eczema: *In vitro* and *in vivo* studies on intestinal microflor. *J Orthomol Med* 5(3):155-157

Kristi: *As of now he has not had any "attacks" for nearly four weeks from mainly adhering to a very strict diet. However, we paid a lab privately who tested for Candida and M. was positive. We then contacted BioCare (Birmingham, England) who gives free nutritional advice about their products and they recommended an Oregano complex which is very high in garlic, along with a digestive enzyme and an artichoke complex that makes the die-off* [of the yeast] *more manageable.*

He will go on to a probiotic and vitamin and mineral supplement in due course. They also recommended drinking as much water as possible - filtered/boiled/bottled. Leaky Gut articles state that with this more natural approach, it can take two years to reach some sort of balance in the gut, and after all, this problem has probably been going on for many years in most patients.

Larry: *I might add many of us have used a combination of many things - before the treatment of fluconazole, my wife was taking a Candida "killer," multiple types of probiotics, grapefruit seed extract, milk thistle and vitamin C.*

Very little research exists for the mentioned supplements other than probiotics, but the Internet is a goldmine of products being promoted and sold. I did find a 2016 review article of N-acetyl cysteine (NAC)[217] stating that NAC is a powerful detoxifying antioxidant supplement as well as a mucolytic drug (meaning it breaks up mucous secretions).

The authors cite studies where NAC is used to treat acetaminophen toxicity, polycystic ovarian syndrome (PCOS), and premature births, infertility, and recurrent miscarriages. They also mention the use of NAC in chronic bronchitis, asthma, Parkinson's disease, and liver cancer.

Other supplements such as turmeric and curcumin are anti-inflammatory and antioxidant. But these products have little research behind them. Of the ones that do, few examined GI or microbiome issues, let alone ABS. So, I say *caveat emptor*; do your homework, because many of these products are just a way to separate you from your money. On the flip side, I won't argue with success.

---

217   Mokhtari V, Afsharian P, Shahhoseini M, et al. (2017) A review on various uses of N-Acetyl Cysteine. *Cell J* 19(1):11-17. DOI: 10.22074/cellj.2016.4872

MEDICAL MARIJUANA

Some ABS patients have tried or are interested in trying marijuana for relief or symptoms. Medical marijuana from *cannabis* plants is now legal now in 34 states, District of Colombia, Guam and U.S. Virgin Islands.[218]

The two sought-after active ingredients are the non-psychoactive cannabidiol (CBD) from hemp (*cannabis sativa)* and tetrahydrocannabinol (THC), the psychoactive ingredient of *cannabis indicus*. The classification of the plant is not as important as measuring the TCH content in any family of *cannabis* plant.[219]

The FDA first approved the cannabinoid, dronabinol (brand names Marinol and Syndros) in 1985 for the treatment of nausea and vomiting. It was especially effective for the nausea caused by chemotherapy and the weight loss associated with AIDS. Later doctors used it to treat anorexia and weight loss in other conditions.

Today CBD is used for seizure disorders and other very serious conditions with an incredibly positive impact. Many patients are also using CBD for anxiety, mood disorders, and pain relief for many ailments.

Several of our patients have used THC to help them with nausea and vomiting during and after a flare. For example, Peter: *I vomit so much, I rarely keep anything down. And then I don't feel like eating. CBD and THC* [components of marijuana] .... *to be honest it's part of the only reason I'm able to get ANY appetite at all!*

I hope many more uses are found as prescribers continue to use this important medication for their patients. For sure, we need studies on the impact of CBD and THC on the gut microbiome and GI disorders.

---

218   National Conference of State Legislatures. State medical marijuana laws. http://www.ncsl.org/research/health/state-medical-marijuana-laws.aspx#3 Retrieved: 6-5-19

219   Ministry of Hemp. Hemp vs. Marijuana. https://ministryofhemp.com/hemp/not-marijuana/ Retrieved: 6-5-19

AROMATHERAPY

Aromatherapy is used in perfumes, cosmetics, and cleaning products for esthetic effect and we all enjoy the pleasant influences to some degree. Clinical aromatherapy, however, is the healing use of essential oils for a desired effect.

A quick search of the academic library retrieves nearly 29,000 peer-reviewed articles on aromatherapy so there's a lot of current science behind the practice. We know that many essential oils have therapeutic traits such as the ability to relax and lessen pain, muscle cramps, and nausea. Other oils have characteristics such as antibacterial, antiviral, and antifungal properties.[220] For example, numerous studies have shown the effective use of tea tree oil or *melaleuca alternifolia* against antibiotic resistant pathogens, including one I co-authored.[221]

I am an internationally certified clinical aromatherapy practitioner and instructor and highly recommend aromatherapy for all of my clients and patients. People with ABS and caregivers can definitely benefit from an individualized plan for healing by a clinical aromatherapist. Please don't just go to a lay person who sells essential oils; find someone who has been trained beyond their healthcare license and practices aromatherapy based on the research.

If you select a book for a personal resource, look for one with credible and recent references. I recommend Dr. Jane Buckle's highly readable 2015 book, *Clinical Aromatherapy: Essential Oils in Healthcare.*

MISCELLANEOUS TREATMENTS

Because I am a Board Certified Advanced Holistic Nurse (AHN-BC [retired]) many people ask me about various integrative and holistic

---

220   Buckle J. (2015) *Clinical Aromatherapy in Healthcare*. St. Louis: Elsevier

221   Chin K, Cordell B. (2013) The effect of tea tree oil (*melaleuca alternifolia*) on wound healing using a dressing model. *The J Compl & Alt Med* 19(12):942-945. https://www.ncbi.nlm.nih.gov/pubmed/23848210

therapies. For therapies I'm not familiar with, I always go to the scientific literature before making a recommendation.

Several of our patients swear by the Rife and Zyto scanners and numerous frequency healing modalities but I was unable to find any research to back the claims. The only published academic articles I found resolutely refuted the machines by saying:

> There is no evidence to suggest that the frequencies Rife claimed to identify are genuine, or that the specific radio frequencies based upon them would kill a retrovirus while leaving host tissue untouched. It is extremely implausible that the low-powered radio frequency Rife machines can have any meaningful biological activity, let alone lethal activity against specific microorganisms.[222]

I caution you to be very careful about untested protocols, supplements, or scanners. Many of these products are just another revenue stream. However, we in the ABS community know all about skepticism and we understand that many scientific breakthroughs come from ideas that were once scorned. Often the ideas are tested first by citizen scientists and then gain credibility through research. So, don't give up if something works for you.

DESPERATE MEASURES

Fecal transplants are a topic of conversation in the ABS support group as a possible treatment avenue for those who have not found relief from the methods mentioned so far. Technically called fecal bacteriotherapy, or fecal microbiota transplants (FMT), fecal transplants are just what they sound like – putting feces from a healthy person's colon into a sick person's colon. I know it sounds ridiculous and certainly rather disgusting but desperate times call for desperate measures!

---

222 The ALS Untangled Group. (2014). ASL Untangled No 23: The Rife machine and retroviruses. *Amyotrophic Lateral Sclerosis and Frontotemporal Degeneration* 15:157–159

When you think of all the illnesses caused by disturbances in the gut, it makes sense that doctors would think of a way to colonize an unhealthy person with healthy microbes. And since no one knows every microbe that makes up a healthy gut microbiome, they have to go right to the source.

Normally, the patient identifies a healthy donor to provide a stool sample, but with the increase in the number of transplants, labs are now preparing donor samples through screening and freezing them. One company, OpenBiome, is providing pre-screened stool samples to over 1,000 institutions.[223] First there were blood banks, then sperm banks, now poop banks! What next?

Most fecal transplants are strictly experimental; however, the Center for Infectious Disease Research and Policy states that new guidelines published on February 15, 2018 included the use of FMT for the treatment of recurrent infections of *Clostridium difficil.*[224] This infection, also known as *c. diff*, is one of the most difficult pathogens causing severe diarrhea and often death and is endemic in U.S. hospitals.

Remember earlier when I wrote about autism spectrum disorder (ASD) being associated with gut dysbiosis? Dae-Wook Kang and other researchers at Arizona State University treated 18 children with ASD using fecal transplants.[225] Multiple data sets were collected before, during, and after the fecal transplants. Sixteen of the 18 patients showed at least an 80% reduction in GI symptoms such as constipation, diarrhea, indigestion, and abdominal pain.

All 18 children with ASD improved on measures of social skills, hyperactivity, aberrant speech, and daily living skills and increased their developmental age by 1.4 years in only eight weeks. Most strikingly, is the strong statistical correlation between GI symptoms and behavior, and the fact that the benefits to the children lasted well beyond the eight-week observation

223   OpenBiome. https://www.openbiome.org/regulatory

224   Dall C. (2018) New C diff guidelines incorporate fecal transplant. http://www.cidrap.umn.edu/news-perspective/2018/02/new-c-diff-guidelines-incorporate-fecal-transplant

225   Kang D, Adams J, Gregory A, et al. (2017) Microbiota Transfer Therapy alters gut ecosystem and improves gastrointestinal and autism symptoms: an open label study. *Microbiome* 5(10):1-16 DOI: https://doi.org/10.1186/s40168-016-0225-7

period. The authors concluded that the protocol is promising for improving GI and behavioral symptoms of ASD.

The Food and Drug Administration (FDA) has yet to regulate FMTs because they have not yet decided if poop is a drug or a human tissue – no joke! Well, it's okay to laugh a little. What is poop? And, is the procedure actually a tissue transplant or just a procedure?[226] These are serious questions the scientists are pondering.

Now I'm going on record to say don't ever try this at home. Please, don't do it! Obviously, some people think that a poop transplant can be done in the comfort of your own home because there are several websites that direct people how to perform a DIY transplant. Seriously though, there are risks of contracting pathogens from each other, risk of tissue damage, and then there's the ick factor, so no at home fecal transplants people, okay?

I'm not aware of a patient with ABS who has had an FMT, but I know that some have considered it in desperation and even discussed it with their doctor. The patient would have to be accepted into a clinical trial and at this time, I'm not aware of any clinical research being done on ABS. Let me know if you hear of any new clinical trials or if someone you know had FMT.

LIFESTYLE

There's clearly no magic bullet for ABS. Managing symptoms of ABS and preventing relapse means embracing a huge shift in lifestyle. Having to give up foods we love like alcohol, ice cream, mashed potatoes, and gravy is difficult enough.

On top of that loss, the ABS patient must confront environmental toxins: external and internal. External toxins include tobacco and nicotine products, molds, fumes, and pollutants. Patients must be especially careful to avoid exposure to triggers and that can be difficult if they want to go out

---

226   Brookshire B. (2018) To regulate fecal transplants, FDA first has to answer a serious question: What is poop? *ScienceNews*. https://www.sciencenews.org/blog/scicurious/fecal-transplants-regulation

in public. Patients may feel their entire life has been upended, their choices stripped away, and that they are no longer safe out there in the world.

Several patients had to change jobs in order to keep flares at a minimum. One patient realized that one of his triggers was the ground coffee he worked around because he was inhaling the dust. He had to quit that job and seek another. Changing jobs is a colossal shift in lifestyle, and for people who are already struggling financially, it feels impossible.

One patient only flared at home when he went to his man-cave in the basement. When his family started investigating, they found mold in the walls of the basement. Once the mold was remediated, his flaring subsided. Still others discovered a larger source of mold in their house and had to move – imagine!

•••••

Internal toxins are the mental and psychological ones: stress, anger, anxiety, frustration, and depression. Because so many ABS patients report flares during periods of stress, including physical and emotional stress, you may find you must incorporate lifestyle changes to help alleviate symptoms and prevent flares and relapse. We all must manage stress in our lives but with ABS you must manage the stress of an illness, and then, even if cured you must learn to manage the stress of your massive lifestyle changes. It's a double or triple whammy.

Not only are you struggling with the physical aftermath of the illness, you are faced with giving up foods you love and alcohol you may have enjoyed. This may have huge social implications of needing to change the way you socialize and maybe even the people you socialize with. You may also find you need to change activity levels, manage anxiety and depression, deal with addiction, and on top of everything, you may experience grief over these losses and changes.

Joe was one of the fortunate ones who took anti-fungal meds, followed a low carbohydrate diet, took probiotics and was cured. He has even been able to return to a more normal diet. But he was also forced to look at his choices and realized he needed to make huge lifestyle changes by implementing exercise, maintaining a healthy weight and diet, abstaining from alcohol, and managing stress through counseling and meditation.

STRESS

Remember when I talked about the effects of the sympathetic nervous response of fight or flight? This amazing response enables us to quickly respond to imminent danger like jumping out of the path of an oncoming car. Unfortunately, the long-term effects of constant levels of being on high alert can result in chronic illness. The differences are summarized in the table:

Fight or Flight Response from Acute Stress	Long-term Effects of Chronic Stress or repeated Acute Stress
• Increased adrenaline • Increased heart rate and breathing • Increased blood pressure • Increased alertness of all senses • Increased cortisol; suppresses GI and immune function; Releases carbohydrates and fat for energy • PTSD	• Fatigue and Sleep Disturbances • Increased appetite and fat storage • Damage to blood vessels and arteries • Chronically elevated blood pressure • Risk for heart attack and stroke • Headaches and digestive issues • Anxiety and Depression • PTSD

Chronic illness, in turn, adds to stress and sets up a vicious cycle. Learning to deal with acute and chronic stress and emotions can be another seismic lifestyle change. You can find hundreds of books and videos (check out YouTube) on stress reduction, but the key is to find something that works for you. Meditation, massage, and yoga are methods with tons of research to show they decrease stress.

Meditation has been around for centuries but in 1979, Dr. Jon Kabat-Zinn developed a therapy for Mindfulness-Based Stress Reduction (MBSR) at the University of Massachusetts combining meditation with yoga. Kabot-Zinn says, "Mindfulness means paying attention in a particular way: on purpose, in the present moment, and non-judgmentally."[227] Numerous other definitions and practices sprang up in the intervening four decades.

A quick search in my academic library revealed over 9,000 scholarly articles on mindfulness in healthcare and 1,153 studies specifically on MBSR. Mindfulness training is used with many medical diagnoses from cancer, multiple sclerosis and diabetes, to mental illness, Parkinson's disease, and PTSD. MBSR is effective in reducing pain, anxiety, and panic attacks.

MBSR is offered in over 200 medical centers, hospitals, and clinics around the world, including some of the leading integrative medical centers such as the Scripps Center for Integrative Medicine and the Duke Center for Integrative Medicine.

Mindfulness is simple to use with training and practice and can be used by anyone, anywhere, even during other activities, such as yoga, running, or cooking. My favorite is mindfulness during daily yoga. If mindfulness can work with the above ailments, it can work for people with ABS.

We still have a lot to learn about lifestyle and treating ABS, so the search continues. But if you are an ABS sufferer, you need to explore the possibilities that work for you. Embrace your situation as an opportunity to discover more about your health. Check out Appendix B for more lifestyle suggestions and tools.

---

227   UMass Medical School. Center for Mindfulness. https://www.umassmed.edu/cfm/

CHAPTER 18   ⟨⟩

THE AFTERMATH

Isolation is at the heart of all disease; therefore, healing requires community and the support of others.

— *Sharon Weil, Author, ChangeAbility*

CURED OR NOT CURED?

Joe believes he is cured. He has not flared for nearly nine years and he eats a healthy diet, abstains from alcohol, and manages stress through exercise; he feels normal. Donato believes he is cured but he and Michelle are more cautious since he's had a couple of relapses and they know that relapse is possible any time he must take antibiotics. For the majority of our patients, ABS has been diagnosed and "cured."

But for several patients, the struggle continues. Nick still experiences relapses even after multiple courses of antifungals. He wrestles with his diet and environment to try to discover the underlying triggers for his flares. He and Karen realize that stress plays a huge role in his flares and he makes big lifestyle changes to reduce his stress. Ray's doctor treated him with common antifungal drugs, but he didn't fully respond. He is still not allowed to travel out of state for treatment because of his legal woes related to the DUI. He grapples with periodic flares.

An overgrowth of yeast was detected somewhere in the intestines of everyone who has been diagnosed with ABS. Most of the patients remember the very course(s) of antibiotics that coincided with the onset of symptoms. But we still wonder at the convergence of factors that led to the constellation of symptoms that induced Auto-Brewery Syndrome. Why does one person get it and not another?

These questions beg to be answered: Is ABS an indication of a more sinister problem such as a genetic mutation? Is it an enzyme deficiency? Is it a genetic predisposition to yeast overgrowth? Is ABS a basic error in the microbiome about which we know so little? Is it something we've done to ourselves through highly processed food, diet, and too many antibiotics? Or is it several of those things?

Whether or not someone with ABS has been "cured," patients and caregivers alike live with the fear that a flare could disrupt their lives again without notice. Relapse is a very real possibility and families must be vigilant in prevention and watchfulness.

RELAPSE OF ABS

Donato was doing well in March of 2018 after his treatment for ABS. However, he had a bout of pancreatitis and went to the hospital. They gave him an IV antibiotic as a "precaution."

Michelle: *On Thursday I met with infectious disease and tried to explain to that doctor about Auto Brewers and how the IV antibiotic they gave him can cause relapse and he could make alcohol from food. She handed me back the newspaper and the business card I had printed with the auto-brewery website and she pretty much blew me off.*

My husband is now back at RUMC in Staten Island, New York, seeing Dr. Jessie and Dr. Das and Dr. Wick's back up, because he is again converting food to alcohol. We are doing the high carb food test and he's brewing, and his sugar is going high again, and we are awaiting the results of his endoscopy cultures.

The message here is this: It doesn't matter if you have ABS or had ABS, as soon as you take an antibiotic you may be back to square one unless the doctor has an action plan to reverse the ABS and kill the yeast. Hopefully we can document a standard protocol for anyone with ABS.

Donato's entire story points out the need for advocacy and an extra dose of assertiveness. Trust me, I know how hard it can be to stand up to doctors who think they know better than their patients. But whether you are the patient or the caregiver, be strong and persist.

ABS AND ALCOHOLISM

In a truly macabre twist, ABS can cause alcohol addiction. Any alcohol is a drug to the body and the near-constant presence of ethanol in one's body causes habituation to the drug whether it's endogenous or ingested. After all the suffering they have endured, ABS patients can become alcohol dependent and must then deal with a new disease - addiction. Not only were many of them dealing with the false accusations of alcohol abuse when ABS first presented, now they are dealing with addiction as a comorbidity.

Thankfully not all, but some of the patients in our group have survived the syndrome and been treated successfully for ABS, only to discover the trauma of alcohol withdrawal with symptoms ranging from mild to devastating. When the withdrawal is overpowering, the body's need for alcohol hijacks the pleasure center of the brain and the urge to drink takes over.

Patient R: *I do want to add one last thing. Once the antifungal medication started to work, I had extreme detox symptoms including shaking, vomiting, and seizures. Because I had ABS for such a long time (I would seem normal at a .25% BAC) I had to check into a detox center and have decided to stay clean and sober.*

Caregiver T: *About 2 months ago, but well after the ABS diagnosis, I discovered my wife was drinking without my knowledge. Hiding it...I caught her three weeks in a row. I essentially said she needed to go to rehab or leave. That was one of the shittiest days I'd had in a long time. She agreed to go. The shakes started within 15 minutes of her getting up. I am giving everyone this information because there is a correlation, in my opinion, with long-term ABS and alcoholism.*

Patient J: *After the ABS discovery, I tried to stop drinking but found the shakes would start so I guess I was self-medicating and one drink became two, and then three and so on...so I would stay intoxicated. It was the only way I could feel better.*

Patients and families need to know that Auto-Brewery Syndrome is real and that it carries a very real risk of alcohol addiction. They also need to know there is hope. A patient must first find a primary provider who believes that ABS exists and is willing to not only treat the ABS, but also help the patient put a plan in place to detox and remain sober when cured from ABS.

Remember that alcoholism is a disease and there are many wonderful treatment resources available from inpatient rehab centers to outpatient counseling. Alcoholics Anonymous is available in every state in the US and nearly every country in the world.

THE IMPORTANCE OF SUPPORT

Haley is a patient and member of the Facebook support group. She illustrates for us the importance of support for patients.

Haley: *For me, I never saw the flares coming. My family and friends notice when I start acting funny. I would check my level with my breathalyzer and sure enough, it would be up; anywhere from .20-.30. I don't remember much during my flares; I usually sleep it off. Once I start to come down, I get really sick – vomiting and a LOT of joint pain.*

I've had many blackouts and my mom tells me that I've fallen a few times because I always try to continue to do things on my own, even though it's obvious I can't. I think as I got more used to the way flares went, I cooperated a little better.

I guess the word I would use to describe the feeling would be "scary." Waking up the following day or later that day, and not remembering anything, getting sick, feeling really foggy for the rest of the day and sometimes even the next day – it's been really scary trying to understand how my body could actually be doing this by itself.

We all need someone to listen to us. Family members express themselves to the group when they are most vulnerable:

Caregiver John: *I was mad, frustrated, at my wit's end. There were several times I was packing up to leave (before I knew it was ABS). I was aggravated that she would 'keep doing this when she knew I would get mad.' What on earth is wrong with her?*

Caregiver Teri: *I felt powerless mostly – that I could do nothing to change the next several hours or days…I knew M. wasn't drinking, but I had no idea what was wrong with him.*

Support is vital for patients and family members to get through every serious illness as well as the aftermath of the illness. When asked if the Facebook support group helped, Donato responded: *Actually, it did. When I was zero, I used to read the posts. Most of the time I didn't post. I just wanted to read them.*

There was a lot of good information out there, and everyone was helping one another. It felt really good that I wasn't alone - I was relieved in one way that I wasn't alone, but it was also encouraging there may be help for me. It's another good support mechanism - but you definitely need friends and family support, too.

And another post: *We didn't do this to ourselves. This was not our fault. We have no control. Get people involved to help you cope - you need friends and family you can trust and talk to so that you can get through this. Don't give up on us.*

CAREGIVERS AND POST-TRAUMATIC STRESS

Caregivers experience a special kind of hell. The chronic worry and stress take a toll. At some point a caregiver may need more support than self, family, friends, or even a group can provide. They may need professional support to cope with the stress of the disease and the aftermath. Here are comments from caregivers posted in the online support group.

Tamela: *I'm so distressed watching Mark slip into a flare with nothing I can do to stop it. I feel frustrated, angry, powerless, hopeless. I feel like nothing we do makes it stop. I can only ride it out and hope his episode is shorter or less severe this time. Everything goes on hold…we don't make plans or reservations or buy tickets anymore because we never know when he'll be functional.*

Molly: *The most painful times are remembering every single moment he could have died; which was every day. Every single 911 call, every flare I watched, every time I watched him struggle for breath and words, every time my friends carried him in my house and helped me put him to bed. The worry when he was out, was that he wouldn't make it home. I re-live every moment.*

Amanda: *He tried to jump out of my car at 60 mph. I've chased him naked through the woods; watched him lying in the road in front of our home, crying in nothing but athletic shorts. I kept his head on my leg to keep him from bashing his head into the concrete while he was thrashing around. I don't think I could ever express all the emotions I've gone through while caring for him.*

Rose: *I've seen my mom struggle so much. Me and my husband do everything we can short of moving in with them to help her. At one point my husband just had to grab her and hold her while she cried. It breaks our hearts at times. I'm so sorry.*

For four years I too lived with frequent bouts of near panic having to deal with Joe when he was in a moribund state. The chronic stress of wondering if today was the day I would watch him die or kill someone else was taxing. I was glad to be a nurse who was trained to handle emergencies but as a wife, the constant tension of frequent flares was exhausting.

The strain of the unknown was a burden that took a physical toll in lost sleep, weight gain, and generalized anxiety. And the fear and pain of not knowing what was wrong with him shredded my heart. I felt completely alone; and I still have flashbacks to the terrifying moments.

I was relieved when he was diagnosed but then I had the added stress of trying to help him find a treatment that would work for him and support him in his lifestyle changes.

Patients and caregivers, but especially the caregivers, continue to live with the aftereffects of the trauma we experienced for the two, five, or even 10-20 years we lived with an unknown, and until recently, untreated condition.

Many of our caregivers describe the symptoms of Post-Traumatic Stress Disorder (PTSD) from the constant fear of our loved-one's death, or the fear of him or her unintentionally hurting someone else. Some also experience the anguish of witnessing the devastating personality changes that can come with intoxication as well as a debilitating illness. The day-to-day stressors accumulate and take not only a physical but also a mental and psychological toll.

Nicole: *I can get easily irritated. Not because a flare could have been avoided but because dealing with a drunk person who has no idea their behavior is off is SO annoying. Especially after years. It's kind of like "Fuck. Here we go again."*

Michelle: *Every day I walked on eggshells. I would silently watch him eat "normal" and be scared to death he would have a positive BAC. I thought once ABS was "cured," some magical veil would be lifted, and I'd get some "ah hah" moment and dance happily in my life, in the sunshine with birds singing. No.*

I have rubber legs, I get shortness of breath, I have chest tightness and I cry - a lot. I make a list and go to the supermarket to get groceries, and I am unable to buy more than one day's worth of meals. I can't think as I walk up and down the aisles. I can't even buy everything on my list. I just buy the bare minimum and say to myself "I'll just come back tomorrow."

I think I can push myself and grab more groceries, but I can't. I want to cry. I have cried, in the supermarket - pushing the cart and having people look at me while tears roll down my face. I don't care that they see me cry. The pain is too great, and it's hard to explain to someone what it was like every day, every minute, every hour. I try and breathe through my panic attacks.

Sometimes I am ok - then I remember something, and I can't breathe. Sometimes when my husband and I disagree, and it gets a little heated, it is a trigger for me - I recall the angry outbursts and behavior when he was having a flare, and I get that tightness in my chest. I withdraw. I shut down. I stop talking. I just can't deal.

● ● ● ● ● ●

As caregivers, we all have days where we are strong and others where we wonder how much longer we can go on. Some report "breakdowns," while others report getting sick or having PTSD symptoms of flashbacks, heart-racing, and difficulty breathing. Many nights after Joe passed out, I used to cry a lot and turn to prayer. During the day I coped by being angry at ABS and often that would come out sideways toward Joe; then I felt guilty. Ugh.

Those of us in the support group remind each other that our feelings are normal. Anger and frustration are normal and it's okay to cry. Those with PTSD lean on the group and may also need professional counseling, pastoral care, or medications. It's okay.

Al-anon is a group for family members or friends of alcoholics and is a great resource. The groups are based on modified principles of AA and can benefit anyone struggling with alcohol-related issues. One couple who went to Al-anon stated that every marriage could use the principles.

Michelle: *My mother tells me "get through the next 15 minutes. Then when you start feeling better, get through the next 30 minutes and so on. Eventually you will be ok." I love my friends & family.*

Karen: *Just a shared thought: My goal the past few weeks has been renewed focus on "me" time and self-care, especially now with additional worries of a close sister diagnosed with stage 3 breast cancer. These tips from Family Caregivers Alliance seem obvious but I recently had to press reset, as I had not known how much I had been slowly sliding away from my own care.*

- *Learn and use stress-reduction techniques (e.g. meditation, prayer, yoga, Tai Chi)*

- *Attend to your own healthcare needs*

- *Get proper rest and nutrition*

- *Exercise regularly, if only for 10 minutes at a time*

- *Identify and acknowledge your feelings, you have a right to ALL of them*

- *Change the negative ways you view situations*

- *Set goals*

- *Take time off without feeling guilty*

- *Participate in pleasant, nurturing activities, such as reading a good book, taking a warm bath*

- *Seek and accept the support of others*

- *Seek supportive counseling when you need it or talk to a trusted counselor, friend, or pastor*

    - *IT'S UP TO YOU!*

    - *Thinking of everyone in the group and wishing you all a relaxing Aloha Friday!*

Caregivers are often the last to take care of ourselves because we are so used to taking care of others especially if they we children living at home. We often feel we don't have time or energy to do anything but care for the person who is ill and manage all the things that make life possible. If you are a friend of a caregiver, offer some respite time: stay with the patient so the caregiver has time for self-care: to be alone or socialize, to exercise or sleep.

And most importantly, reinforce the idea that it's not only okay, but necessary for caregivers to take care of ourselves and ask for help if we need it. Some may need professional counseling or medication to get through the illness and aftermath. Please take care of yourselves.

CHAPTER 19 ～

THE FUTURE

I think I might tell my children in 10 years that the early 2010s was a barbaric era.

— Bertalan Mesko, The Guide to the Future of Medicine: Technology AND The Human Touch

I do not know the future, but if I use history as a guide, here are some of my speculations about the destiny of Auto-Brewery Syndrome. ABS will follow the convoluted progression of many syndromes and other chronic ailments related to the microbiome. Not in linear fashion, but in overlapping fits and starts.

Providers will continue to deny ABS but gradually consider it. More people suffering from symptoms will band together to share information. Citizen scientists will continue to advocate for recognition, diagnosis, and treatment. More and more providers will hear about it and realize it's a real syndrome. Lastly medical researchers, in due time, will target ABS for study and find better treatments.

The list of mystery diseases without medical consensus for diagnosis and treatment is endless with new ones emerging every year. We know that ABS, like IBD and IBS, are strongly linked to disturbances in the gut micro-biome. These diseases followed a convoluted history of discovering causes and treatments. For centuries IBD and IBS were premature.

Not until the 1950s did science catch up to these ailments. Because these are relatively common disorders (10-15% for IBS and 4% for IBD), support groups around the world have raised money for extensive research and clinical trials. Even though the etiology and cure are still unknown, technology is improving diagnosis and treatment by leaps and bounds.

Chronic Fatigue Syndrome is another elusive disease connected to the microbiome. According to the Mayo Clinic, theories for the cause of chronic fatigue syndrome range from viral or yeast infections in the gut to stress.[228] In the past, doctors blamed hysteria or confabulation for many diseases with unknown causes. Much like addiction, these chronic and rare diseases still carry the stigma of being psychosomatic or "all in your head."

As mentioned earlier, even multiple sclerosis, cystic fibrosis, diabetes, and ASD are now linked to a disturbance in the microbiome. I believe the more we learn about the gut microbiome, the better we'll be able to understand and treat all these mentioned diseases and especially ABS.

HOPE

We're depending on the history of these diseases to light the way for Auto-Brewery Syndrome. Our cause for hope for ABS is that while scientists are still debating the cause of IBS, IBD, and chronic fatigue syndrome, at least they are recognized in the literature by prestigious medical institutions.

Remember the discussion of SIDS and phantom limb in Chapter 1? Those stories of scotoma and their recognition give us more cause for hope. Even when the cause of SIDS was unknown, scientists continued to search for answers until they developed a working hypothesis and they continue to search for answers.[229] And while the scotoma of phantom limb was forgotten numerous times and was scientifically premature, finally scientists believed it and firmly established that knowledge in the medical treatment of amputations.

228   Mayo Clinic. Chronic Fatigue Syndrome. https://www.mayoclinic.org/disease-conditions/chronic-fatigue-syndrome/symptoms-causes/syc-20360490 Retrieved: 1-14-19

229   McEntire B. (2018) National SIDS Act of 1974. https://sids.org/about-us/sids-historical-perspective/ Retrieved: 6-5-18

We only need a handful of researchers to champion ABS. New developments in microbiology, genetics, immunity, and pathology are progressing at lightning speeds. Information technology will revolutionize the science of the microbiome and finally include the mycobiome and virome. New powerful treatment technologies are being developed to deal with many diseases at an astonishing rate.

Epigenetics promises a great impact on obscure or difficult diseases such as ABS. Epigenetics is the modification of gene expression to prevent disease rather than altering the genetic code itself. Since we don't know if there are genetic contributors to ABS, we hope researchers will delve into the genes of people who suffer from ABS, especially those who continue to relapse.

Sequencing technology and bioinformatics are already transforming our understanding of treatment methodology. According to two translational geneticists, Drs. Holger Heyn and Manel Esteller, the future of medicine is to individualize lists of genes to combine conventional treatments with novel drugs to customize treatments.[230] If our patients could get drugs, nutrition, and supplements that are tailor-made to their gut microbiomes, treatments could be shorter and have fewer side effects. That would be amazing!

Many of our patients and caregivers have great hope in holistic therapies. We have tried many of them ourselves and know they work. We believe that trial and error will show more options for integrative treatment and eventually the science will catch up to the modalities that work.

I also have great hope because of our ABS citizen scientists who advocate daily by educating physicians, medical groups, nursing organizations, researchers, and legal experts. Our advocates provide published case studies, research, information, and personal stories to try and get the word out about ABS. This was the year ABS was finally recognized and added to one list of rare diseases.

---

230   Heyn H, Esteller M. (2012) DNA methylation profiling in the clinic: Applications and challenges. *Nature Reviews: Genetics* 15:679-692

ACTIVISM

Compassion is an unstable emotion. It needs to be translated into action, or it withers.

— Susan Sontag, Regarding the Pain of Others

A chronic disease begets compassion fatigue. It's easy to rally around a patient who has surgery and is back in action after 10 days to six weeks; it's more difficult when the patient is sick with an unknown illness for years. Frustration and anger seep into our lives, friends drift away, relationships end. We must channel our feelings into something positive, or we'll go berserk.

Sufferers and caregivers champion many "difficult to diagnose" or rare diseases into medical consciousness. Such diseases dodge easy diagnosis because they often include a host of chronic symptoms such as headaches, fatigue, and muscle aches. Mainstream medicine doesn't address these common symptoms with any consistent treatment other than pain medications or anti-depressants.

It's a tough pill to swallow that with all the technology we have available today, there are still diseases without known causes or cures. Medicine is slow to adapt, and often healing does not even feel like the primary objective. Have you ever felt like a doctor prescribed medicine just because he or she didn't know what else to do? Medicine is still messy, and at best an educated guess, but patients and caregivers continue to push scientists to search for true causes and effective integrative treatments.

I believe we will find multiple factors contribute to the syndrome rather than just a handful of pathogens. Medicine may not always stand on the latest scientific information, but as an eternal optimist, I believe science will ultimately prevail.

What is certain in my mind is that advocacy - those incredible and wonderful citizen scientists that I have the professional and personal satisfaction of working with - will push the envelope in getting providers to listen to us. We continue to share our stories and spread education.

Michelle: *Once we received a confirmed diagnosis, we had to find a treatment. EVERY DOCTOR TURNED US AWAY. Every major hospital in Manhattan and nearby locations had no clue- never heard of this.*

How did we get a doctor and cure? Simple: I became the biggest, persistent, professional, courteous pain the ass, and I NEVER accepted no as an answer. NEVER. That did not mean that I did not accept being turned away. I did. I did not want to fight with an egotistical doctor who did not believe us. I also respected those doctors that were honest and admitted they did not know what to do. I kindly asked them to start researching this, as ABS is in their wheelhouse.

Armed with information, I was able to talk in a professional, courteous manner, and collaborate with doctors to help us. That took us many phone calls, and doctor visits almost EVERY DAY. We were turned away by all but one doctor. But ONE doctor is what you need. Just that ONE.

Here is Michelle helping another ABS patient after an Emergency Room (ER) visit*: S. had gone to the ER, and as expected the ER never heard of ABS. S. was treated for alcohol withdrawal symptoms and discharged.*

I faxed the case studies, with my open letter to the attention of the doctor. The very next day the doctor from the ER called me and wanted to know why I had sent this to his attention, and wanted to know more about ABS. I explained to him that he had taken care of a patient that was suffering from alcohol withdrawal but did not drink and explained we are trying to bring awareness to doctors.

I explained that there IS a way to test if a person has ABS. Although he may not have remembered the patient that he treated in the ER, he thanked me for sending him the case studies. He said he was not even aware that this condition existed! He said that he would do more research on this and learn more about it - as this was the first time he heard about ABS, and he thanked me.

I want that future – with doctors like that and an advocate like Michelle!

······

We need to spread the word beyond the healthcare community as well. Jane was a police officer for over 20 years. She was taught to be aware that some people with diabetes can appear and act intoxicated but might really be experiencing acute ketoacidosis due to their disease. She only discovered ABS when a loved one was admitted to the ER with a BAC of .40 when they knew he had nothing to drink.

Jane: *Knowing what I know now, I wonder how many people we may have sent to jail who might have been telling the truth about not consuming alcohol.*

I remember how angry I would get when they would deny drinking when I was standing there at the van with the "truth" staring me in my face. In a large metropolitan medical center, I can imagine how many "drunks" they must see in a day's time and how angry the doctors must feel when confronted with that same denial when the "proof" of a high BAC is staring them in the face, too.

Like I was, these medical professionals are ignorant. We ALL need to be educated about ABS, just as I was informed about the diabetes problem way back in 1978.

That is why this site [Facebook support group] *and the sharing of information is SO important. I yak about ABS to anyone who will listen. Some of the people say, "That doesn't even make any sense. Are you sure about that?" Other times they are curious and open to learning more about it.*

I was very angry with the doctors who treated us so badly at first, even though we were giving them all of the information about ABS we could get our hands on. Now I realize that they were and still are, acting out of ignorance.

Some may never come around, the ones who think that the MD after their name stands for "minor deity" and their judgment must never be questioned. Others, like the doctor we are seeing now, turn themselves inside-side-out to help us find answers. We are all still learning. It is only through knowledge that we gain power over whatever comes to us in life that just doesn't "make sense."

All our citizen scientists continue to work behind the scenes on this awareness campaign. Stacey and Larry continue to study and share information in the support group. Michelle and Donato advocate and share their story with doctors and medical organizations wherever they can.

Ray and Sierra feel compelled to "shout from the rooftops," until the legal world will listen and recognize an ABS diagnosis. Nick and Karen have been very open and outspoken in telling their story to media outlets in hopes of educating others. Believe me, we all appreciate the media coverage of this hidden disease, including television shows such as Royal Pains, Grey's Anatomy, and The Resident that use ABS as part of their story lines. Thank you and keep them coming!

ABS is a scotoma, but we will no longer let it be forgotten or denied. I know our citizen scientists will continue to spread the word to skeptics and challenge the status quo.

I'M TALKING TO YOU

Joe and I are grateful that he is doing so well after nearly nine years; he's healthier overall now than he was then, and he has no symptoms of ABS, but Auto-Brewery Syndrome has changed my life in more ways than I can count. I continue to rely on the ABS support group for strength and courage to challenge the power structure in medicine.

Initially, I was angry at the disease, frustrated with Joe, and most certainly furious with the majority of the medical establishment that shunned us; How could people who took the Hippocratic Oath inflict such harm? I've spoken throughout this book about providers who denigrate, blame, and shame victims of illness; and I've called on them to be more open-minded, compassionate, and caring. No wonder people turn to holistic practitioners.

Now I'm talking to you. This entire book is a call to action. I've put everything I know about this scotoma called Auto-Brewery Syndrome into this book with an expectation that you the readers will help spread the information. This way our Syndrome will no longer be ignored, denied, or forgotten.

I'm asking you to talk about ABS, educate others, and spread the word. I'm asking all of us to stop judging people who are ill whether they are ill with ABS, the horrible disease of alcoholism or any other health issue. Inside and outside the hospital, we need to treat sick people the way we want to be treated. Please join us in becoming an advocate to put care back in healthcare.

······

THE BURDEN AND THE GIFT

When I was twenty years old, I wrote in my journal "Blessed are the enlightened for their road is fraught with burdens." Knowledge is power. As a society we value education because we believe that science improves lives. But just like the terrible discovery of Auto-Brewery Syndrome, that power comes with a burden; a responsibility to use our knowledge for good.

Auto-Brewery Syndrome dropped in my lap; Joe and I didn't ask for it. But knowing about ABS carries the burden of sharing that knowledge. Once we understand ABS, we have a duty to advocate on behalf of patients, family members, and friends. We must ask people to take it seriously. We need to shout it from the rooftops. We must demand that healthcare providers listen to us, read the science and treat patients appropriately.

On the other hand, ABS is a gift. In the long run, caring for someone with ABS made me a better nurse advocate, a better observer, and a better communicator. It also made me a better wife; I recommitted to Joe "in sickness and in health." Our experience took me deep into my scientific nature which always takes me deep into my holistic essence as well. I'm awed by the human body in health let alone in surviving a disease. And for all that I am grateful.

Our bodies are wonderfully made. We are more microbe than human, and the microbes are what nurture us, protect and defend us, allow us to feel deeply, and shape our minds. But those microbes that usually live in harmony can turn on us too. Disease points out how delicate the balance of our health really is and urges us on to more important questions about holistic health, our diet, our environment and how to maintain that balance.

There never seems to be an endpoint to our scientific and holistic discoveries and health is no exception. Stay tuned for the next chapter in the chronicle of Auto-Brewery Syndrome.

ABS SYMPTOMS/TRIGGERS AND POSSIBLE LINKS

Symptoms/Triggers	Chemistry/Biochemistry	Possible Link
Gut Fermentation from eating or drinking: • Carbohydrates • various sugars – some high fructose corn syrup, some simple sugar, some fruit, etc. • Alcohol sugar of any kind (esp. wine or beer)	Yeast overgrowth: *Candida albicans, Candida krusei, Candida glabrata, and Candida kefyr, with Saccharomyces cerevisiae* seeming to be the most virulent - as evidence by our sickest and most intractable patients.[231] Welch also found *Candida glabrata* in their case study.[232] *Candida Parapsilosis, C. Intermedia.*[233] Earlier studies identified *Candida tropicalis, Candida fukuoka, Candida guilliermondii, Candida stelloidea, Torulopsis glabrata.*[234]	Gut dysbiosis (from antibiotics, leaky gut, etc) Genetic predisposition? Enzyme deficiency or mutation? ADH? ALDH?

231   Cordell B. Kanodia A. (2016) Auto-brewery as an emerging syndrome: Three Representative Case Studies. *Journal of Clinical and Medical Case Reports* 2(2):5. https://doi.org/10.13188/2332-4120.1000013

232   Welch B, Prabhu N, Walkoff L, Trenkner S. (2016) Auto-Brewery Syndrome in the setting of long-standing Crohn's disease: A case report and review of literature. *J Crohn's & Colitis* DOI: https://doi.org/10.1093/ecco-jcc/jjw098

233   Ahmed S, Wickremesinghe P, Kopetz V, Sarkar S. (2018) A rare diagnosis of Gut Fermentation Syndrome/Auto-Brewery Syndrome in the setting of diabetes and obesity. *American J Clin Path* 150:S2. https://doi.org/10.1093/ajcp/aqy090.003

234   Kaji H, Asunuma Y, Yahara O, et al. (1984) Intragastrointestinal Gut Fermentation Syndrome: Report of Two Cases and Review of Literature. *J Foren Sci Soc* 24(5):461-471

Flares caused by eating or drinking Sugar-free products Artificial sweeteners (aspartame,* sucralose, acesulfame)	Aspartame ingested breaks down into its three constituent components: phenylalanine, aspartate, and **methanol** Aspartame is blamed for many health problems, including headaches, seizures, chronic fatigue syndrome, memory loss, and dizziness. It has also been associated with an increase in multiple sclerosis, Alzheimer's disease, and cancer. [235] The Environmental Protection Agency set a recommended limit of only 7.8 milligrams per day of methanol, while a one-liter aspartame-sweetened beverage contains about 56 milligrams, or eight times the recommended amount.[236]	Genetic error in processing phenylalanine (maybe a form of intolerance) or methanol Change in gut bacteria Metabolic syndrome?
Flares from other activities • Stress • Skipping meals • Physical work	Body trying to compensate Low blood sugar	

235 https://science.howstuffworks.com/innovation/edible-innovations/artificial-sweetener6.htm

236 https://www.scientificamerican.com/article/artificial-sweeteners-may-change-our-gut-bacteria-in-dangerous-ways/

Extreme BAC readings (i.e. >.30)	Ingredients include:	Acetaldehyde?
• Snuff, dip, chew • Mold • Other: Unknown	• Arsenic: a poison used in insecticides, rat poison, and anchoring cement in houses • Cyanide: a poison found in chemical weapons and car exhaust • Polonium 210: a highly radioactive and chemically toxic element found in nuclear waste • N-Nitrosamines: cancer causing toxins also found in brake fluid and granite countertop cleaners • Nicotine, an addictive drug	

	• Formaldehyde: a cancer-causing chemical found in glue and gas stoves. Preservative for corpses • Cadmium: found in batteries, motor oil and gear oil • Cyanide, a poisonous compound • Arsenic, a poisonous metallic element • Benzene: found in unleaded gasoline, car engine degreasers, insecticides, motor oil and paint • Lead: a nerve poison found in high-mileage motor oil and ceramic glaze • Uranium 235: a toxic chemical also found in nuclear weapons such as the atomic bomb.[237],[238]	Formaldehyde

237   American Academy of Otolaryngology. (2018) https://www.entnet.org//content/smokeless-tobacco

238   Know What You Are Chewing. https://www.guardyourhealth.com/health-topics/tobacco-free/tobacco-ingredients/

Solvents (glue and paint removers)	Solvent Ingredients may include:	Byproducts or additives: Acetone, xylene, turpentine, toluene, methanol and ethanol
	• dichloromethane, also called methylene chloride, which has serious health risks including death • orange oil or other terpene solvents • N-methylpyrolidone, esters such as dibasic esters • aromatic hydrocarbons • dimethylformamide • Nitromethane • Dimethyl sulfoxide [239],[240]	
Air Pollution	Emissions from ethanol-containing gasoline [241] • Ethanol • Acetaldehyde	Acetaldehyde and other byproducts
Caustic paint removers	Caustic paint removers, typically sodium hydroxide (also known as lye or caustic soda), work by breaking down the chemical bonds of the paint by hydrolysis	Byproducts: Ammonia

239   U.S. Consumer Product Safety Commission. (2013): https://www.cpsc.gov/Global/Safety%20 Education/Home-Appliances-Maintenance-Structure/423%20Paint%20Stripper%20Publication.pdf

240   United States Department of Labor. OSHA (2018). https://www.osha.gov/SLTC/ methylenechloride/

241   Suarez-Bertoa R, Zardini A, Kueken H, Astorga C. (2015) Impact of ethanol containing gasoline blends on emissions from a flex-fuel vehicle tested over the Worldwide Harmonized Light duty Text Cycle (WLTC). Fuel 143:173-182. http://dx.doi.org/10.1016/j.fuel.2014.10.076

Grain dust, mold spores	Carbohydrates and/or mold Chaetomium is fungi that can produce mycotoxins that cause poisoning [242] Myxomycetes are slime mold-like fungi	Inhalation
High or Low Blood Sugar issues/ Fermentation flare	Possible compensatory/ interference mechanism by yeast interacting with insulin and/or glucose stores	Unknown

242   Mold Sickness (2018). http://moldvictim.org/mycotoxins/

CHECKLIST IF YOU MIGHT HAVE ABS

Pre-Diagnosis

1. Keep a logbook or journal that includes everything you put in your mouth: food, drink, tobacco, gum, candy, medications, etc. Be specific.

2. The second column in your logbook should be for activity and location: physical work, workouts, sleep, exposure to environmental toxins like mold, smoke, fumes, etc. and where you are – especially when you have a flare

3. The third column in your logbook is for symptoms, mood and feelings: nausea, tiredness, stress, lethargy, confusion, active, happy, etc.

4. The fourth column in your logbook is for alcohol readings from your breathalyzer

5. Document everything in your logbook throughout the day with as much detail as possible. Allow a caregiver to help you remember items you may overlook

Pre-Diagnosis Breathalyzer

1. Purchase a Department of Transportation (DOT) approved breathalyzer

2. Cost is around $100 or more. Well-known brands include BACTrack, SafeWay, and AlcoHAWK

3. Use the breathalyzer throughout the day and record the readings in your logbook

4. Allow a caregiver to assist you if you are experiencing symptoms

Diagnosis: Finding a Doctor

1. Visit the website: www.autobrewery.info and see if there is a treating provider near you. Look under "Resources"

2. Find an open-minded gastroenterologist, infectious disease practitioner, or primary provider who can perform tests to diagnose other underlying issues such as SIBO, gastroparesis, etc.

3. Some patients recommend asking the provider to test for intestinal yeast overgrowth rather than ABS since so many healthcare providers have never heard of ABS. Show them your logbook

4. If at first, you don't succeed, try, try again! Keep pushing to get diagnosed

5. Ask your provider to call Dr. Wick listed on our website since his group will assist other doctors willing to follow their protocol

Diagnosis: Confirming ABS

1. The diagnostician should review your logbook and take a detailed history

2. You may wish to have a 24-hour observation to confirm endogenous alcohol production with blood draws, not just a breathalyzer. This can be done in a hospital or out-patient with someone monitoring access to alcohol.

3. The observation can be done to prove to a skeptical doctor, employer, family member, or even yourself, just wanting confirmation

4. Request Breath testing to diagnose other underlying conditions. Especially look for delayed transit time or gastroparesis

5. The doctor should order an EGD and colonoscopy to collect samples from the stomach, small intestine, and colon to identify the contributing yeast. They must request a DNA identification of the yeast

6. You and your provider may also decide to have you tested for food allergies since ABS can mimic food allergies and sensitivities

Treatment of ABS: Flares, Medication, and Diet

1. Stay safe! Treat alcohol poisoning as it happens. High readings can be very dangerous, and you may need medical treatment

2. Once diagnosed, you have a right to choose the course of your treatment from conventional or holistic treatments or a combination of methods anywhere on the spectrum.

3. Conventional treatments include a range of antifungal medicines. Your provider will help you choose based on the culture, yeast ID, and your response to medication

4. Diet is a very important part of any treatment and will include a low carbohydrate eating plan.

5. Review your logbook to assess your personal food triggers and avoid them when possible.

6. If no relief, try an elimination diet, adding back foods one at a time to assess those that trigger a flare

7. Consult a nutritionist for help with your decisions and any compliance issues

8. Abstain from alcohol, permanently

9. Consider taking probiotics, either recommended by a provider or on your own. Be sure to choose a probiotic, either as pill or food, with live organisms, a diversity or microbes, and high levels (in the trillions)

10. Collaborate with providers and request referrals when needed

Treatment of ABS: Lifestyle

1. Review your logbook to identify internal (stress, frustration, anger, etc.) and external environmental triggers (location, mold, allergens, tobacco use, exposure to toxins, etc.) for flares

2. Take an unvarnished look at your lifestyle and where and how you can make changes. What triggers can you eliminate or avoid? Do you need to stop using tobacco?

3. Change activity levels (more exercise? Less screen time?)

4. Implement stress reduction (yoga, massage, meditation, prayer, talking with friends?)

5. Beware of unproven modalities that just separate you from your money

6. Focus on the positive things in your life and get counseling if you need it. It's okay to ask for help

7. Choose what works for you! You are in charge!

Care for Patients and Caregivers: Stress Reduction

1. Practice Mindfulness (go to a website or get a book and learn the basics): https://www.umassmed.edu/cfm/mindfulness-based-programs/mbsr-courses/

2. Do yoga, take a walk, cook, be active

3. Pamper yourself

    a. Get away

    b. Get a massage

    c. Listen to music

    d. Knit

    e. Color

    f. Be creative

    g. Do something just for you – EVERY day!

8. Join a support group

9. Ask for help if you need it

10. Get counseling

ACKNOWLEDGEMENTS ～

First and foremost, I'm grateful to my husband Joe. He was my first ABS patient, and the first case study I published. Initially, he wanted to remain anonymous but over time he began to tell his side of the story. Joe baby, I love you and I would have done anything to help you get well. You were the inspiration for all the research, articles, and now this book.

You put up with hundreds of hours of me with my nose buried in the computer answering emails, developing the website, participating in the support group, and of course finding and reading every book and article I could, that might shed light on abnormal gut fermentation. I'm so happy you're well and I love it when you cook dinner for us. Thanks a million, my honey!

The book would not be nearly as interesting without family members and patients willing to tell their stories. Karen and Nick, Michelle and Donato, Larry and Stacey, Sierra and Ray – you are the ones that will help so many others by telling your incredible true stories. Thank you for trusting me with your most intimate details of this horrific illness called Auto-Brewery Syndrome. Our stories are the ones being shared and I hope I have treated them with the care and attention they deserve.

And then there are the doctors: I can't emphasize enough how humbled I am by open-minded doctors willing to listen to patients with ALL their senses, suspend disbelief, act like a scientist, search the literature, and call a nurse an expert! The most important one in my healing circle is Dr. Justin McCarthy. When Joe was sick, you listened to us with an open mind, even if your eyes were widened.

You read the stack of articles I gave to you and ran all sorts of tests and tried the treatments described in the literature. You even consulted with me along the way and suggested we write up Joe's case for publication because it was unique and there was so little in the literature. You are the best doctor in every way.

I know there are more providers out there, but the other main ones we know of are Dr. Anup Kanodia, Dr. Wickremesinghe, Dr. Das, and Dr. Jesse Saverimutti. You are the way all doctors should be! Thank you.

Appreciation goes to attorney Joe Marusak for reviewing the story of the ABS patient he represented; ensuring its accuracy and adding a few previously unpublished details. I appreciate all the other caregivers and patients who shared in the support group and allowed me to share their experiences and words.

Susan Rushing, my dear friend and mentor, was helping me search the internet and literature and first hit on the term "Auto-Brewery" when Joe was hospitalized in ICU for one of many times. Thank you, Susan, for your support and brilliant mind; otherwise Joe and I (and many others) might still be in the dark about what the heck was causing those bizarre symptoms.

Immense gratitude goes to the librarians at Panola College in Carthage, TX, especially Sherri Baker. Sherri, you spent untold hours searching for articles that became my scientific references. You were invaluable in finding obscure journal articles, chapters in books, and even recommending references you thought I needed. You are a gem.

Warm appreciation to scientist Jeff Leach and his amazing work on the American Gut Project. Your inspirational publications such as *Rewild* and others kept me on the path of this harrowing journey called Auto-Brewery Syndrome. The American Gut Project was also very forthcoming with data and questions we used in our research and for that I am grateful.

A big shout out to Michaeleen Doucleff of National Public Radio (NPR) for her article "Auto-Brewery Syndrome: Apparently You Can Make Beer in Your Gut" for the Salt blog in 2013 (https://www.npr.org/sections/thesalt/2013/09/17/223345977/auto-brewery-syndrome-apparently-you-can-make-beer-in-your-gut). You put my article on the worldwide map and it resulted in over 54,000 downloads in 2013-14 alone. You started me on this path to answering emails and calls, creating a website, an appearance on ABC's 20/20, BBC and made me even more determined to find answers. So, thank you, Michaeleen wherever you are.

Very importantly, the recognition in the media has directed over 500 people my way who were suffering symptoms of Auto-Brewery, with over 250 of them receiving a diagnosis of Auto-Brewery Syndrome. Without journalists and reporters, the ABS sufferers would not have found me and kept me motivated. Thanks to media outlets everywhere including NPR, CNN, BBC, Clear Channel Radio, local TV stations, and others that called to find out more about ABS. Freedom of the press is essential to a thriving democracy - Write on!

Last but not least, my gratitude goes to my writer/editor friends who inspired me and read versions of the book with kind and loving feedback. Jane Webb-Childress, my friend and first run editor, you are appreciated for your time and feedback, and making corrections with your "teacher pen." You have taught me so much about reading and writing over the years for which I am grateful.

While the book might have been written, it never would have been published without my amazing and wonderful everything editor Miranda Culp. You helped me organize and express all my feelings along with the messy science. You helped me find my critical voice and vent my anger without being too harsh; and of course, you encouraged me to inject a little humor into a subject that doesn't lend itself to much laughter. The words "thank you" are not enough for what a big job you had on your hands with me and my nerdy science that I love. You helped me go from an academic writer to a "real writer." I am blown away by the result and will be eternally grateful. You are the best!